T0331994

OXFORD STUDIES IN ANALYTIC THEOLOGY

Series Editors
Michael C. Rea   Oliver D. Crisp

OXFORD STUDIES IN ANALYTIC THEOLOGY

Analytic Theology utilizes the tools and methods of contemporary analytic philosophy for the purposes of constructive Christian theology, paying attention to the Christian tradition and development of doctrine. This innovative series of studies showcases high-quality, cutting-edge research in this area, in monographs and symposia.

The Contradictory Christ

JC BEALL

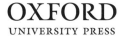

OXFORD
UNIVERSITY PRESS

OXFORD
UNIVERSITY PRESS

Great Clarendon Street, Oxford, OX2 6DP,
United Kingdom

Oxford University Press is a department of the University of Oxford.
It furthers the University's objective of excellence in research, scholarship,
and education by publishing worldwide. Oxford is a registered trade mark of
Oxford University Press in the UK and in certain other countries

First Edition published in 2021

Impression: 2

Published in the United States of America by Oxford University Press
198 Madison Avenue, New York, NY 10016, United States of America

British Library Cataloguing in Publication Data
Data available

Library of Congress Control Number: 2020951048

ISBN 978–0–19–885236–0

DOI: 10.1093/oso/9780198852360.001.0001

Printed in Great Britain by Bell & Bain Ltd, Glasgow

For all who've sensed the contradiction, and to any who've yet to do so...

Preface

Aim

This book has one aim: to advance a contradictory christology – and thereby a contradictory christian theology – as concisely as possible compatible with user-friendliness, and with an emphasis on the big picture rather than intricate details. As such, the book does not answer all details that academic theologians or philosophers or biblical scholars may raise; future discussion enjoys an invitation from the future. The point of the current work is to put the account in broader conversations beyond academic journals. (This isn't to say that the book is a 'trade book' – it isn't – or that it's written with an eye specifically on the mythical 'general reader', but the book is written without pausing at every potential academic concern.)

Previous work

Substantial parts of this material were first published in *The Journal of Analytic Theology* (JAT) as a symposium on my initial definition and defense of Contradictory Christology (Beall, 2019*a*). Despite the overlap, this book presents significant new aspects of the account, including positive reasons for accepting the account, comparative comments on salient alternatives, a handful of new objections and replies, and a brief glimpse towards future work on a unified approach towards the trinity.

Future work

This book focuses on christology, and in particular the so-called fundamental problem of christology (much more on which throughout the book), namely, the apparent contradiction of Christ's being fully human and fully divine. The book is intended to be the first in a two-book series (of sorts), the second focusing in depth on the trinity. The final chapter of this book (viz., §6) sketches a few – but only a very few – preliminary issues in the directions of subsequent work.

Hope

My hope is that readers who are at least not dogmatically committed to the standard off-the-shelf story of logic (viz., so-called classical logic) find this book to be not only interesting but illuminating – perhaps even liberating, loosening one not from the demands of a rational christian theology but from the demands of a logically consistent one, allowing one to shake off the scales and accept the inconsistent truth in its scandalous but awesome glory.

I carry no illusion of final achievement in this work. Elements of the full truth, we know not exactly which ones, are vastly beyond us. But as responsible, systematic thinkers we are obliged to give the true and complete-as-possible account, to the best of our abilities. This book is a step in that direction. By my lights, the true theory of Christ is inconsistent: it contains contradictions, claims that are false but, critically, also true. Conveying at least that much is my hope.

Target audience

The target audience is genuinely interdisciplinary (and 'transdisciplinary' and so on); it's a very broad and varied audience. This book is written in a way that is intended to be accessible to both theologians and philosophers; however, the book chiefly aims to make a theological contribution, written and read by theologians who are not only interested in how best to make sense of the apparent contradiction of Christ, but are also interested in the pursuit of systematic theology as a systematic truth-seeking enterprise, an enterprise thereby subject to the universal constraints of logic and the space of logical possibility.

Conventions governing style

Religious names and adjectives: spelling. While its rationale remains unclear to me I nonetheless follow standard English convention in using uppercase

'C', 'J', and 'M' when talking about Christians, Jews, and Muslims, understood as those who, respectively, accept target christian doctrine (for my purposes, doctrine and creeds affirmed at least up through the Council of Chalcedon in 451), jewish doctrine, and islamic doctrine. In turn, and as reflected in the previous sentence, I use lowercase letters when the target terms are in adjectival position. One rationale for this is simply aesthetic. Scattering a multitude of uppercase letters all over a Page makes for Aesthetically displeasing Pages. Another rationale is that my chosen convention is in keeping with related conventions, including the common observation that one can be a Platonist without spending one's life dreaming of platonic essences or engaging in platonic relations or even endorsing all platonic doctrines. The same considerations apply to christological theories (any christology), which are systematic accounts of Christ. If a specific christology is under discussion, such as Conciliar Christology (per Timothy Pawl's work) or even Contradictory Christology as specifically developed in this book, uppercase letters may be used – but even here, I admit, there's very strong pressure against the uppercase.

Quotation marks. I use single quotation marks in what, at least in phi-losophy, is often called the *Analysis* convention. On this convention, single quotation marks are used in three very different ways, where the given usage is always clear from context. First, I generally use single quotation marks to mention words, as when I mention the word 'mention'. I also use single quotation marks for direct quotation, as when I directly quote Professor Dr. Oliver Crisp who, in conversation, once replied to something I said by saying nothing more nor less than 'Very good.' (The only exception to the direct-quotation convention is exceedingly rare: viz., a direct quotation within a direct quotation within a direct quotation. This is so rare that further comment on the convention is unnecessary.) Finally, I use single quotation marks for scare quotes or (equivalently) shudder quotes, as when I say that enjoyable 'pains' might not be pains at all. As always, communication rests largely on context, and when it comes to quotation conventions context is the cure. And if one wants a rationale for adhering to the given *Analysis* convention, I turn to two rationales. First, once again, there is an aesthetic one: single quotation marks do the job without cluttering pages. Second is Ockham-ish: why use more marks when fewer will do?

Em dashes. Here again, I follow the given *Analysis* style by spelling an em dash as an en dash flanked by the single-space character – as I do in this sentence. (The other, perhaps more common, way of spelling em dashes does so without spaces—as done in this parenthetical remark.) The *Analysis* spelling is cleaner; it uses less ink; and most important is that it's aesthetically more pleasing, at least by my lights. Since both spellings of the em dash do the trick, I use the cleaner, less-ink-using and aesthetically more pleasing one.

Displaying or labeling/listing sentences. I often either mention (occasionally use) sentences by either displaying them, as in

> This sentence is displayed.

or labeling or listing them, as in

1. Some sentence is true.
A14. Some tractors are green.
CD. Some trees are green like some tractors.

Always (except, perhaps, in this initial example), context makes plain what's going on – whether the sentences are merely mentioned for some reason, or whether they're mentioned for purposes of labeling, but then either used in some way (e.g., indirectly used via ascribing truth to the sentence so labelled) or just mentioned by way of their new tags. The reason I'm highlighting this convention is not that it's unfamiliar or requires explanation; I'm highlighting the convention to explain another convention used a lot in the book. The target convention concerns use of labels. In particular, I refer to (1) – the first sentence above labeled by the numeral '1' followed by a period (the full-stop dot) – by '(1)' but refer to A14 and CD just so – no parentheses required. The difference is that the numeral '1', much like the full-stop dot (the period), has a very standard use in English while neither 'A14' nor 'CD' do. The latter tags are always interpreted per the given context of use; the numeral for the number one and, likewise, the full-stop dot are always interpreted per their standard and widespread meanings unless the context otherwise makes the matter abundantly clear. Of course, there may be an argument to the effect that flanking 'A14' and 'CD' with parentheses unifies the target convention with the parentheses flanking '1' in '(1)'. That's true, but here again is where aesthetics – and general ease on the eyes – swims to the surface: why clutter the page with further marks when none would do? The unifies-convention argument doesn't tip the scales.

Chapter relativity of labels. There is one more convention related to using labels for sentences: namely, that if sentences are enumerated using standard numerals, such as (1) above, the label is chapter-relative. If one were to flip through subsequent chapters and see '(1)' in the pages, one would be mistaken to think that (1) above – in the preface (viz., 'Some sentence is true') – is being discussed. The convention requires that one stay within the chapter and look for the explicit introduction of the label '(1)' in that chapter, and the sentence so labelled is the sentence being discussed.

Chapters, subchapters, etc. Except in this preface, reference to chapters, subchapters, etc. are almost always given by '§' followed by the target number, so that '§2' refers to Chapter 2, '§2.1' refers to Section 1 of Chapter 2, and so on: the first numeral following '§' is the chapter, the second (if a second) the section in said chapter, the third (if a third) the subsection, and so on.

Authors and their work. I refer to an author (e.g., Richard Cross) and a piece of the author's work when I truly say, for example, that Cross (2011) gives a succinct but highly illuminating and equally influential discussion of the fundamental problem of christology – the fundamental problem confronting the core christian doctrine of the incarnation. Here, 'Cross' in 'Cross (2011)' denotes Cross while the parenthetical item denotes the given work, namely (and here is another convention), Cross 2011. When an author's (sur-/last/family) name immediately precedes a numeral (usually, the name of a year) or a numeral-cum-letter (e.g., '2020*a*' or the like) – separated only by one occurrence of the space character (viz., ' ') – the resulting expression is being used to denote the given author's work, not the author, so that, as above, 'Cross 2011' denotes only Cross' given work, not Cross. In short, 'Cross (2011)' denotes both Richard Cross and also Cross 2011, but 'Cross 2011' denotes only Cross' given work, namely, Cross 2011. Similarly, when parentheses enclose a comma flanked by an author's name and the name of a year (with or without an alphabetical subscript), such as '(Cross, 2011)', the entire expression – parentheses and all – refers to the work and only the work. A similar convention applies when multiple works are cited, except that semicolons are used to separate target items, as in '(Coakley, 2002; Cross, 2011; McCall, 2015; Pawl, 2016; Rea, 2003; Stump, 2003)'.

An unsolicited note on reading the book

The chapters are ordered, more or less, in a typical dependency series. There's one exception. §2 of this book talks about logical consequence ('logic', for short), its role in true theories (and, hence, in the true theology), and what, by my lights, is the correct account of logical consequence. Despite my efforts to make §2 a user-friendly, from-scratch presentation, some readers who've never studied the mainstream account of logical consequence may find §2 to be a very-low-gear chapter. If you are such a reader, my advice is to read §2 for the big ideas, and slide past the details. Subsequent chapters can be mostly understood without an understanding of all details in §2. (Mostly. There are a few technical issues in subsequent chapters that turn on technicalities of the given account of logic, but they are not mandatory for the central ideas in the book.) The core theses of the book can be understood without having full competence of the given account of logical consequence.

Acknowledgments

Mike Rea and *Sam Newlands*: they've been genuinely invaluable resources for the project from early on. Both have shaped the resulting account more than they know. They are not only extraordinary philosophers; they are generous in their engagement. During (too?) many Notre Dame Center for Philosophy of Religion (CPR) seminars on my work, Newlands often defended my position against Rea's objections better than I did. I just took notes. Without their help and encouragement, this project simply wouldn't've been completed – full stop.

Tim Pawl: Pawl's work on christology shows up a lot in this book, not because it's true, and not just because it's false, but because it's now one of the front-running candidates in the long-running quest for a consistent christology. Pawl, from day one, has been a generous interlocutor, a fierce critic, and a steady, reliable source of extremely dry – think hot, crushing, desert-like – humor.

A. J. Cotnoir: Cotnoir remains a source of philosophical and theological ideas. Without his help this project either would be worse or wouldn't be at all.

Oliver Crisp: his work sparked many of my own thoughts on many topics in this book. Moreover, Crisp's generous interaction with me while we were CPR fellows at Notre Dame – and especially at 'high table' dinners together – was enormously helpful.

Andrew Torrance: his engagement with my work during a 2019 visit to *Logos* in St Andrews was extraordinarily helpful, not only in forcing clarity of my views but in exposing me to Torrance's own incipient explorations along the lines of 'paradoxical theology'.

JAT Symposiasts: In addition to Cotnoir and Pawl (above), both Thomas McCall and Sara Uckelman generously engaged with my work in a *Journal of Analytic Theology* symposium on my initial position paper (Beall, 2019a). These four thinkers deserve special thanks not only for pointing to apparent problems but for providing the encouragement to fix the problems.

2018–19 fellows at the Notre Dame Center for Philosophy of Religion: Kimberley Kroll, Dawn Eschenauer Chow, Meghan D. Page, Patrick Kain, and, once again, Oliver Crisp were wonderful colleagues at Notre Dame's CPR.

Their generous but severely critical feedback proved to be tremendously helpful, even more useful than weekly vegan outings to India Garden.

Late-draft feedback: I'm grateful to Mitchell Mallary for extensive feedback that improved the final draft, and also to Joshua Cockayne, Justin Harrison Duff, Matthew Joss, Vi Bui, and Jonathan Rutledge for late-draft comments.

Indexing and comments: Joseph Lurie deserves special thanks not only for feedback on a late draft but for doing much of the indexing for the book.

Four others whose influence has been very strong: *Richard Cross*, in his work and in our occasional correspondence, remains an invaluable source for my thinking on the target topic(s). In addition to Cross I should again mention *Thomas McCall's* work; it introduced me to analytic theology, and his comments have pushed the work in important directions that I wouldn't've otherwise considered. I am also very grateful to *Susana Gómez*, who provided enormous encouragement and inspiration in many ways, not only in her own work but also in conversation. Lastly in this context, but in no way least, I happily acknowledge *Philip-Neri Reese, OP*, who provided tremendously insightful criticisms of my contradictory theology; I remain very grateful for the time and effort that he invested early on.

In addition to the people mentioned above, there are some philosophers who have been particularly helpful over the years in discussing ideas that have fed this book. Before listing the others one stands out: namely, *Graham Priest*. As references throughout the book reflect, Priest was an early advocate of contradictory theories; his career has been a steady force in search of gluts (i.e., 'true contradictions'). My work, on the other hand, has long been much (much) more conservative than Priest's, with my work reflecting next to no gluts – not none, but next to none. Still, without his work and without our many conversations and collaborative projects over the last twenty years, this work would likely not be what it is – in fact, it most definitely wouldn't be.

Others with whom I've discussed elements of this project are Donald Baxter, Rebecca Brewster Stevenson, Laura Frances Callahan, Colin Caret, Dustin Crummett, Franca D'Agostini, Rasa Davidaviciute, Natalja Deng, C. Daniel Dolson, Sean Ebels-Duggan, Elena Ficara, Patrick Greenough, Jared Henderson, Grace Hibshman, Justus Hibshman, Dominic Hyde, Mengyu Hu, Thomas Hofweber, Andrew Jaeger, Nathan Kellen, David Lincicum, Bill Lycan, Stephen Ogden, Hitoshi Omori, Colin McCullough-Benner, Chris Mortensen, Daniel Nolan, Martin Pleitz, Stephen Read, Greg Restall, David Ripley, Gillian Russell, Jeremy Sakovich, Sharon Southwell, Andrew Tedder, John Troyer, Zach Weber, and Nicole Wyatt.

Administrative help: Joyce Zurawski of Notre Dame provided seamlessly efficient administrative help during early stages of this project. Her competence and efficiency allowed me to focus on the book project without needing even to blink over critical administrative issues.

Copyright/overlap: per Preface, substantial parts of this book were published in *The Journal of Analytic Theology* as a symposium on my initial paper on the topic (Beall, 2019a). My hope is that even those who've carefully and exhaustively read the symposium will find that this book better illuminates the overall account and answers key questions left hanging in said symposium.

Institutional acknowledgement: I'm grateful to both the University of Connecticut and the University of Notre Dame for research support, and likewise to UNAM's Institute for Philosophy, Melbourne University, and both the *Logos Institute* and *Arché Centre* at the University of St Andrews.

Finally, I'm grateful to Katrina Higgins for being who she is.

Jc Beall
Notre Dame

Contents

THE WORD BECAME FLESH AND MADE HIS DWELLING AMONG US.
John 1:14

... BOTH MAN AND GOD: ON THE ONE HAND BORN, ON THE
OTHER NOT BORN: ON THE ONE HAND FLESHLY, ON THE OTHER
SPIRITUAL: ON THE ONE HAND WEAK, ON THE OTHER EXCEED-
INGLY STRONG: ON THE ONE HAND DYING, ON THE OTHER LIV-
ING. THAT THESE TWO SETS OF ATTRIBUTES, THE DIVINE AND
THE HUMAN, ARE EACH KEPT DISTINCT FROM THE OTHER, IS
OF COURSE ACCOUNTED FOR BY THE EQUAL VERITY OF EACH
NATURE.

Tertullian, Treatise on the Incarnation (trans. Evans 1956)

[THE] ONE LORD JESUS CHRIST, THE SON OF GOD, BEGOTTEN
FROM THE FATHER ... TRUE GOD FROM TRUE GOD, OF ONE
ESSENCE WITH THE FATHER, ... WHO BECAUSE OF US HUMANS
AND BECAUSE OF OUR SALVATION CAME DOWN AND BECAME
INCARNATE, BECOMING MAN, SUFFERED AND ROSE AGAIN ON
THE THIRD DAY ... *The Nicene Creed*

... OUR LORD JESUS CHRIST IS ... ONE AND THE SAME SON, THE
SELF-SAME PERFECT IN GODHEAD, THE SELF-SAME PERFECT
IN HUMANITY; TRULY GOD AND TRULY MAN ... ONE AND THE
SAME CHRIST, SON, LORD, ONLY-BEGOTTEN, RECOGNIZED IN
TWO NATURES, WITHOUT CONFUSION, WITHOUT CHANGE, WITH-
OUT DIVISION, WITHOUT SEPARATION; THE DISTINCTION OF
NATURES BEING IN NO WAY ANNULLED BY THE UNION, BUT
RATHER THE CHARACTERISTICS OF EACH NATURE BEING PRE-
SERVED AND COMING TOGETHER TO FORM ONE PERSON AND
SUBSISTENCE, NOT AS PARTED OR SEPARATED INTO TWO PER-
SONS, BUT ONE AND THE SAME SON AND ONLY-BEGOTTEN GOD,
THE WORD, LORD, JESUS CHRIST ...

Chalcedon 451

1

Contradictory Christology

In this chapter I present the principal thesis in a concise, big-picture way. Subsequent chapters fill in more details.

1.1 The longstanding christological quest

The familiar christological quest is a quest to 'consistentize' – to give a consistent account of – Christ. For a flavor of the familiar quest, think of Jews and Muslims and any other religious or religiously inclined non-christian informed thinkers. Think even of early Christians.

- At first, Jesus is seen as just another human person.
- ... and then some see him as a very wise human person.
- ... and then some see him eventually as a prophet, in line with past prophets.
- ... and then some see him even as the long-promised messiah – *the christ*.
- *But see him – the walking, talking, sweating Christ Jesus – as God?!*

Here, even when one recovers from the shock of a seemingly blasphemous and clearly scandalous suggestion, incredulity quickly sets in:

- A GodMan doesn't even make sense! Christ Jesus is human. How can Christ Jesus also be divine?
- The very idea is nonsense, sparking contradictions at every turn ...

... And then, as if from the wilderness, a voice cries out:

- ... ahh, but Christ Jesus' being God is not contradictory if Christ Jesus is not really a human, and hence not a human person at all ...

The Contradictory Christ. Jc Beall, Oxford University Press (2021). © Jc Beall.
DOI: 10.1093/oso/9780198852360.003.0001

And so goes what we all know as the longstanding quest to consistentize Christ. Other voices steadily follow the first but in different directions:

- ... ahh, and it's not contradictory if there are really two persons involved in Christ Jesus, the human person Jesus and the divine person Christ ...

... and yet other voices:

- ... ahh, and it's not contradictory if Christ Jesus is neither a god nor a human but instead has some hybrid nature overlapping with but different from God's nature and different from our nature ...

... and so on, including:

- ... ahh, and it's not contradictory if the predicates true of Christ Jesus (e.g., 'divine', 'human', etc.) are not really the same predicates they appear to be – they mean something different from how we standardly use them.

... and so on. And there are many, many more voices crying out, each trying in ever-elaborate ways to advance a contradiction-free account of Christ.

In the end, I've come to think that the response of non-christian thinkers is more telling than the many consistency questers have noticed. The long-standing charge from informed non-christian thinkers (both theists and non-theists alike) is familiar: *that Christ is both the one and only god (viz., God) and is as human as any human* is either contradictory or nonsensical. The latter horn should be rejected: the claim clearly has sense (meaning); it's precisely the scandalous and jarring sense that sharpens the first horn, and scandalous and jarring meaning is meaning all the same. It's along these lines that non-christian thinkers appear to have long seen the apparent truth of Christ. By my lights, it's time to accept the truth as it appears: contradictory.

And it isn't just non-christian thinkers who see the apparent contradiction. Reflective, truth-seeking Christians have sensed the contradiction too, and they have twisted and squirmed to avoid it: witness the long parade of heresies (e.g., only partly divine but fully human; only apparently human but fully divine; and so on and so on and so on and so on ... and on ...), each an attempt to explicitly avoid the contradiction, each part of the ongoing quest to consistentize Christ.

The quest to consistentize Christ – the quest to give a consistent solution to what Richard Cross (2011) famously dubbed 'the fundamental problem of christology' – enjoys a long, fascinating history; and the quest continues in full force up through today. But I believe that the quest should end. I believe that christian thinkers should accept the contradiction of Christ.

1.2 The central thesis: Christ the contradiction

Christ is a contradictory being. So goes the central thesis of this book. At the crux of christian theology is a contradiction: namely, Christ Jesus is a being of whom some claims are both true and false. That's it.

That some claims are both true and false of Christ is not a claim involving new meanings of 'true' or 'false'. Likewise, that some claims are both true and false of Christ is not a (so to speak) kenotic or partial or degree-theoretic claim; it's not a disguised way of saying that some claim is (say) partly true but fully false of Christ or, the other way, fully true but partly false of Christ. The simple thesis of this book is that some claims are both true and false of Christ – full stop, no new meanings, no playing with words.

A witness to the contradictory truth of Christ is the familiar conclusion of the familiar fundamental problem of christology (Cross, 2011):

1. Christ is human. [Given]
2. Christ is divine. [Given]
3. Christ is mutable. [1: human nature entails mutability]
4. Christ is immutable. [2: divine nature entails immutability]

So, by logic, (3) and (4) entail that Christ is both mutable and immutable. But, at least on standard usage, 'mutable' and 'immutable' express *contrary properties*. Contrary properties are ones that are jointly had only at the cost of contradiction. And the target contradiction is manifest to many: it's true that Christ is mutable (because Christ is human) but it's false that Christ is mutable (because Christ is divine). And this is but one of many (many) such contradictions entailed by Christ's two-natured being – by the incarnation of God, one person both fully human and fully divine.

The fundamental problem of christology is simple to see. On orthodox or standard christian theory – by which I mean Chalcedon-constrained christology (viz., Council of Chalcedon I at 451) – Christ is the divine, omniscient God who, with all humans, exemplifies human nature with its innumerable limitations, including imperfect knowledge, imperfect understanding, and so on.[1] The apparent contradiction is vivid, fueled by the foundational role of Christ in orthodox christianity. An omniscient being could not have our imperfect understanding of the pains and frustrations of our limited epistemic states unless – and here is the problem in a nutshell – the being were not omniscient. The apparent contradiction fuels the pull of the kenotic tradition in christology which, against orthodox christianity (my principal focus throughout), puts priority on exactly one of the two natures. The pull of kenotic christology arises from the simple contradiction of, on one hand, Christ's needing to be imperfect (limited, etc.) in order to have the experience of imperfect (limited, etc.) agents, but, on the other hand, Christ's being God and thereby without imperfections (limitations, etc.).

The fundamental 'problem' of christology is simple to see from the role that Christ occupies: the Christ figure is to have the divine and essentially limitless properties of the one and only God (i.e., properties that impose no limits on God beyond logical limits) but Christ is equally – and not in some watered-down fashion – to have the human, essentially limit-imposing properties involved in human nature, limits essentially involved in being human just like you and me.[2] The role that Christ occupies thereby appears to demand a contradiction: all of the limitlessness of God, and all of the limits of humans. The way that this contradiction is achieved – the way that Christ realizes the apparently contradictory role – is exactly as the standard (Chalcedonian) account seems to imply: the having of two contrary natures, the one divine and the other human. Conciliar texts within standard christian tradition use language like 'passible and impassible' and 'capable of suffering and incapable of suffering' (Tanner, 1990, p. 162), but the explicit contradiction comes quickly from plain paraphrases of such standard terms (e.g., 'incapable' as 'not capable' etc.).

On the christology being advanced in this book, Christ plays the foundational role of having all of the features required to fully experience suffering

---

[1] My claims about Chalcedon are not intended as the end point of the careful historical analysis and interpretation reflected in the work of, for but two examples, Anatolios (2011) and Daley (2018); however, my claims throughout are intended to reflect the very real apparent contradictions with which the long history of christian thought, from historical to philosophical to theological to pastoral perspectives, continues to grapple.

[2] One should never forget that even if divine nature and human nature have similar properties but in importantly different degrees (e.g., omniscience versus partial knowledge, etc.), the limits on each human-nature property are firmly capped (so to speak); otherwise, we humans could be just as unlimited as God, which requires some possibility in which we humans *are* as unlimited as God – and this is deeply against the grain of standard christian doctrine, so much so that, by my lights, it counts as an absurdity in the true theology.

exactly as we experience it while at the exact same time being worthy of worship (not just worthy of respect, not just worthy of reverence, but worthy of *worship*) and incapable – not capable – of such suffering or imperfect understanding of such suffering. The contradiction of Christ, on the proposed christology, arises not because of sloppy thinking by christian thinkers; it arises because Christ's foundational role in christian theology requires something contradictory – and thereby something extraordinary, unique, and awesome. Of course, if logic itself required that a contradiction – the logical conjunction of a sentence and its logical negation – entails outright absurdity, then the central thesis of my account would be absurd and immediately off the table. But logic itself (i.e., the correct view of logical consequence) doesn't rule it out – an issue to which §2 is devoted (viz., the question of *how* the account avoids logical absurdity). And so the question is whether the apparent contradiction of Christ is veridical, of whether the true christology is logically inconsistent – an issue to which §3 is devoted (viz., the question of *why* the account should be accepted over the standard consistency-clinging accounts).

Christians have long embraced the radicalness of the incarnation, not as something fashionably radical (say, 'far-out' or 'cool' or 'woke' or whathaveyou) but rather as deeply, soberly, fundamentally radical, cutting to the very warp and woof of reality, the union of the divine and the human into neither two persons nor a new hybrid nature but rather as just what the incarnation is: the one and only God who is a divine person (in that he is divine and he is a person), who is a human person (in that he is a human and he is a person), and whose striking being is foolishness by normal, mainstream standards. The properties essential to such a radical being contradict one another: unchangeable but changeable, perfect but imperfect, able to sin but unable to sin, all-knowing but ignorant, and on and on and on and on and...with contradictions enfleshed by the being whose role demands nothing less.

There is but one god (viz., God), most holy, perfect, and unchanging in such qualities; and to claim of a human – as human as you and me – that he is precisely the one and only god (viz., God) is to either fool around with the usage of words or to land in apparent contradiction. Confrontation with such apparent contradiction immediately but erroneously elicits poetic interpretation of the claim, mere analogy, figures of speech. The central thesis of this book is rather that the apparent contradictions are true – full stop, no poetic license involved, no analogical buffers required. The incarnation doctrine, which is by all lights radical and difficult to believe, is apparently contradictory, just as non-theists and traditional non-christian monotheists have long said. But the contradiction is true. That's the central thesis.

1.3 Terminology: contradiction and contradictory beings

A *formal contradiction* is any sentence of the form

> it is true that . . . and it is false that . . . .

where both ellipses are replaced by the same sentence, and where 'it is true that', 'it is false that', and the given 'and' are logic's truth operator (sometimes called 'null operator' or 'nullation'), logic's falsity operator (often called 'logical negation') and logic's conjunction operator (often called 'logical conjunction'), respectively.[3] In turn, a *contradiction* is any sentence that entails a formal contradiction.

A *contradictory being*, as discussed above, is a being of whom some contradiction (per above) is true.

Terminological note on contradictory beings: for simplicity and convenience, if a being is a contradictory being (as above), I often say that the being is a contradiction, even though, strictly speaking, contradictions are as above – namely, sentences of the form *it is true that . . . and it is false that . . . .*

Terminological note on paradox: The term 'paradox' is sometimes used in many different ways in theology. If 'paradox' were used to mean nothing more nor less than what 'contradiction' means then my central thesis would be equivalent to a rewording involving 'paradox'. But the term usually means something importantly different from (oftentimes less than) what 'contradiction' means. In particular, 'paradox' is often used in a way that essentially involves some sort of epistemological status – something to do with how much we can know or truly believe or the like. Paradoxes, on common usage, are *apparent contradictions*, that is, claims that appear (to a theorist or observer etc.) to entail contradictions. Contradictions are different. A contradiction is a contradiction regardless of how it appears to us. To only call Christ a 'paradox' may be true (given said usage), but it is misleading if, as I claim, Christ is a contradiction, as misleading as it would be to say only

---

[3] All so-called pieces of logical vocabulary, together with an account of logical consequence itself, are presented in §2.

that Christ apparently hung on the cross. For the most part, I avoid the term 'paradox' in this work, as 'contradiction' cuts to the central truth.[4]

1.4 The rarity of true contradictory theories

To ward off a concern from the start, let me make something perfectly plain: I am not hereby proposing that theologians should seek to find contradictions willy nilly. The reason that we generally reject all logical contradictions is that true ones are ultimately few and far between. And this is why so few of our true theories are contradictory. As §2 discusses at much greater length, logically possible contradictions are ruled out in many theories as theoretically impossible, given the nature of the theory's target phenomenon. Standard mathematics rules out – or blocks off – the logical possibility of contradictions as *mathematically* impossible; and much of physical theory, biological theory, many metaphysical theories do the same. But in strange cases of extraordinary phenomena the full truth requires a contradiction.

My proposal is not that theologians ought to seek out contradictions; the proposal is that Christ's unique role motivates a contradictory account – his exemplification of two contrary (contradiction-entailing) natures. Having the two contrary natures brings about the truths entailed by having the one nature and the falsehoods of having the other (and vice versa, the truths of the other and the falsehoods of the one): it's true that Christ is mutable (because Christ is human) and it's false that Christ is mutable (because Christ is God). Said together just so is jarring; but such is Christ's role in the christian worldview. As a methodological principle, we should not seek out contradictions but we should be open to the rare cases that motivate them.

---

[4] I'm grateful to Andrew Torrance and Josh Cockayne for prompting the foregoing clarification on 'paradox' versus 'contradiction'. I should also note that I am resisting an explicit comparison of my view with projects specifically under the flag of 'paradoxical theology', as discussed by Torrance (2020) and Evans (1989). Kierkegaard is a paradigm of such 'paradoxical theology', but while, by my lights, Kierkegaard recorded many truths about the incarnation, much of his writing is subject to hermeneutical guesswork, including whether, for example, his words should be taken as *his* words. And I'm very much not expert on the requisite hermeneutics of Kierkegaard's work. I think it better that I make my own position as clear and precise as possible, and herein invite experts on 'paradoxical theology' to flag important overlaps between that project (or family of projects) and my own work. I remain very interested to learn of any such important overlaps (if any). The closest I come in this book to an explicit discussion of something that may be similar to the paradoxical-theology project is in §4 and §5, where I discuss the work of Anderson (2007).

The having of two contrary natures is one case that appears to motivate a contradictory theory, notably, a contradictory christology.

Consider an analogy with Truth and Falsity. These are contrary properties in the sense that having them both entails a contradiction. Were there to be some entity that exemplifies *both* of these properties the entity would be a rare one, something surprising – though perhaps not properly mysterious. As discussed in §2, I maintain that a very respectable – and, indeed, correct – view of logic is that logic itself does not rule out such an entity, something that is both true and false. Logical consequence (logical entailment) enjoys its role of being universal and topic-neutral by being very rich in the possibilities that it recognizes. (Logic's role as universal and topic-neutral entailment is elaborated in §2.) As it turns out, there are entities – admittedly strange and rare – that apparently instantiate or exemplify or have both of the given contrary properties. Witness the familiar and ancient Liar paradox:

✓ The ticked sentence is false.

This sentence is both true and false if it's either true or false. While logic itself won't force the issue,[5] the ticked sentence is a live candidate for the very rare case in which the contrary properties of truth and falsity are exhibited together. As systematic theorists (including systematic theologians) we have a methodological goal of resolving as many claims into the true and the false as possible. Logic, on my view, doesn't demand as much, but systematic theorizing motivates the methodological goal. And with that goal, one is quickly motivated to the view that the ticked sentence is false and also true.[6]

It is important to emphasize that the ticked sentence is a strange and unexpected case. Moreover, by accepting that the ticked sentence is a surprising case of an entity that exemplifies contrary properties, we are not thereby committed to accepting that all peculiar sentences are truly contradictory.

---

[5] In order for logic itself to force the issue one needs something like the law of excluded middle, which is not valid according to the account of logic (viz., FDE) that I advance in §2, and have discussed elsewhere (Beall, 2017, 2018).

[6] That a true theory of these sorts of peculiar entities (the Liar sentence or similar property/set sentences) might be contradictory is an idea discussed by many, including Asenjo (1966); Asenjo and Tamburino (1975), Beall (2004, 2009), Dunn (1966, 1976), Priest (1979, 2006), Routley (1979), Routley and Meyer (1976), and many others, though Priest's work has championed and defended the view more than any other work on the topic. Indeed, Priest's philosophical career and large body of work, much like the late Sylvan's (née Routley) career and work, has focused largely on advocating and defending the spread of contradictory theories beyond this limited area. (This has very much not been my own approach, which has been – and remains – very conservative with respect to accepting the actuality or even theoretical possibility of contradictory entities.)

The very nature of the ticked sentence – a twisted prima facie contradiction – motivates a contradictory theory of it; but few other sentences are like that.

And the same is true of the vastly more important case of Christ: his role is prima facie contradictory; his realization of the role via contrary natures reinforces the contradiction. Indeed, when one asks how something could realize a contradiction, orthodox christology has provided a clear and deeply fascinating answer: namely, the having of two contrary natures. In the end, when the truth is laid bare, Christ may be the unique contradictory being in reality. That's for future discovery to tell. For now, Contradictory Christology, as I advance it, affirms the apparently contradictory orthodox christology as genuinely contradictory. It is true that Christ is mutable; it is false that Christ is mutable. This is jarring, and even in some ways mysterious, but orthodox Christianity has advanced the role of Christ to be just so: jarring and in various ways mysterious. In this case, the mystery, at least in part, is that there is a being whose very existence entails contradictions – that he is perfect and all-knowing but is imperfect and has limited knowledge, and so on for the many other contrary properties true of Christ.

1.5 Summary and looking forward

'What's the thesis?' is the topic of this chapter. The central answer is that Christ is a contradictory being, a being of whom some contradictions are true. More details are given in subsequent chapters.

An urgent question arises in response to the central thesis. The urgent question is: *How does the thesis avoid incoherence?* The question is pressing in the face of one tremendously large tenet in theology: namely, that *logic itself rules out 'true contradictions'.* Since logic is universally binding, applying to true theories if any, the apparent absurdity and/or incoherence of any would-be true contradictory christology is plain.

How, then, is the apparent absurdity avoided? Details are in §2. The short answer is that the alleged absurdity rests on a mistaken view of logic itself. Agreed: logic is universal in applying to all true theories, and so applying to the true theology. Likewise agreed: true theology is bound by the space of logical possibility: any theological possibility is a logical possibility. But the critical point of disagreement: there are no logical possibilities in which some sentence is both true and false (a so-called glutty possibility) – a true contradiction – and there is no logical possibility in which some sentence is neither true nor false (a so-called gappy possibility).[7] By my lights, logic itself recognizes glutty and gappy possibilities; these are both logical possibilities (i.e., possibilities as far as logical consequence goes). Logic is generous with respect to the possible relations that a sentence can have with respect to the fundamental truth values – Truth and Falsity (or, if you like, The True and The False). In particular, unlike the mainstream account (viz., so-called classical logic), which says that logic recognizes only the familiar two combinations (labeled 't' and 'f')

t : sentence A only has value Truth; it's just-true
f : sentence A only has value Falsity; it's just-false

a better (and, by my lights, the correct) account of logic is one according to which logic recognizes the other two combinations too:

b : sentence A has *both* Truth and Falsity; it's a 'glut' of Truth and Falsity
n : sentence A has *neither* Truth nor Falsity; it's a 'gap' of Truth and Falsity.[8]

Possibility b (for '*both* true and false') is directly relevant to the proposed contradictory christology; it's the one wherein both a sentence and its negation (and, hence, their logical conjunction) are true.

Such glutty options have been entirely ignored by theologians for a very long time. But theologians aren't alone. Many systematic theorists concerned with truth and logic have largely adopted the mainstream account – the so-called classical-logic account – of logical consequence (i.e., the relation of *what logically follows from what*). This practice is understandable, since many

---

[7] The terminology 'glutty' comes from 'truth-value glut', where these are sentences that are both true and false (and, so, in some sense have a 'glut of truth values'). The terminology was first used by Kit Fine (1975). The dual of a glut is a gap, where 'gappy' comes from 'truth-value gap', where these are sentences that are neither true nor false (and, so, in some sense fall into a 'gap of truth values'). The mainstream account of logic (i.e., of logical consequence) recognizes neither glutty nor gappy logical possibilities. §2 discusses these ideas at greater length.

[8] Such terminology can also be expressed as follows:

t : sentence A is related *only* to The True (just-true); A only has value Truth
f : sentence A is related *only* to The False (just-false); A only has value Falsity
b : sentence A is related to *both* The True and The False (glutty); A has Truth and Falsity
n : sentence A is related to *neither* The True nor The False (gappy); A has neither Truth nor Falsity.

Thanks to Mike Rea for prompting me to give both ways of talking – where both are intended to be equivalent here (at least for purposes at hand).

phenomena seem to be truly and fully described by theories whose space of possibilities is simply the space recognized by classical logic. But the narrow mainstream account of logic is ultimately built on sand.

That the mainstream view is built on sand is clear: the account was constructed as an account of logical constraints in true mathematics – and only true mathematics. Of course, as an account of the logical constraints in true mathematics, the mainstream account of logical consequence gets things right (at least by my lights). But an account of logical consequence *in mathematics* is one thing; an account of logical consequence – of the logical constraints across *all true theories* – is something else. Why think that the correct account of logical consequence in mathematics, wherein many of our common terms ('truth', 'God', 'adult', and other such vague terms, etc.) are removed from the language, is the correct account of logical consequence *simpliciter* – the correct account of logical consequence for the full, rich language we speak, for all true theories and their respective languages (including, again, the language of theology)? By my lights, there is no good argument for thinking as much.

A better account of logical consequence (simpliciter), one built on stone, is one that recognizes all four of the combinations around Truth and Falsity (viz., as above, the options tagged as t, f, b, and n). There is an account along these lines (viz., so-called FDE for 'first-degree entailment') that enjoys exactly the same truth and falsity conditions for the logical vocabulary as the mainstream (viz., so-called classical) account. In this way, the meanings of logical vocabulary are what they've always been; it's just that some theories (e.g., true mathematics, many of the true scientific theories, etc.) restrict the space of logical possibilities, ruling out logic's glutty and gappy possibilities as theoretical impossibilities. Moreover, there's a simple argument for this stone-founded account. Details aside, the argument is that we lose no true theories and we gain highly valuable – and I think true – theories of at least very strange phenomena, the greatest of which is the scandalously boundary-breaking Christ, who appears on the surface to demand contradictions in the union of contrary divine and human properties.

There is much more to say by way of details. That is the job of §2 and subsequent chapters. For now, my rough answer to the pressing question concerning logical coherence (avoiding logical absurdity) is plain: Contradictory Christology, as I advance it, agrees that logic is universal (applying to true theology just as it applies to true physics etc.), but the mainstream account of logic that governs much of systematic theology is mistakenly narrow. Logic allows for possibilities that go beyond the usual (mainstream-recognized) two; it allows for both gluts and gaps. The contradiction who is Christ exemplifies some of logic's glutty possibilities. Since such possibilities are recognized by logic, the driving worry about logical absurdity or incoherence is simply misplaced.

2

Logic and its possibilities

The two assertions 'Christ is a man' and 'Christ is God' are
prima facie opposed to one another. It seems impossible that they
should both be true; and this impossibility is apparently a logical
impossibility.

– (Williams, 1968, 515)

Per §1 the central thesis of this book is that the full truth (i.e., the complete
true theory) of God incarnate contains contradictions, claims that are true
and false – specifically, claims that are true and false of Christ, the GodMan.
On the mainstream view, both in theology and in philosophy, every contradiction is logically absurd in the sense that any contradiction logically
entails every claim whatsoever, including that Christ is Satan, that 1+1=5,
that Martin Luther was (literally) an heirloom tomato, that Mother Teresa is
best known for her work in advanced mathematics, and every other untruth.
That the true christology (ergo, the true theology) contains contradictions
flies in the face of the mainstream view of logic. But the mainstream view of
logic is not – and has never been – stamped by the authority of revelation
or official doctrine of the catholic (small 'c') church.[1] The mainstream view
persists mostly by unreflective, dogmatic practice, a practice that can and

---

[1] During a Notre Dame workshop on an early version of this book, Thomas McCall observed
that the Catholic church, at least in Vatican 1 on 'Faith and Reason', says things that look like
it's officially stamping a family of accounts of logic (of which the mainstream account is one).
Vatican 1, in Session III under Canons on Faith and Reason, says:

> God cannot deny himself, nor can truth ever be in opposition to truth. The appear-
> ance of this kind of specious contradiction is chiefly due to the fact that either the
> dogmas of faith are not understood and explained in accordance with the mind of
> the church, or unsound views are mistaken for the conclusions of reason.

Of course, I agree that God cannot reject the truth of God's existence. Moreover, I agree that
truth can never be opposed to – and can never in any way undermine – truth. But all of this
is compatible with a rejection of the mainstream view of logical consequence, and indeed an
acceptance of the logical possibility of gluts (or, dual, gaps). After all, even in the case of a glut (a
truth which is also false), the truth is true – and it's in absolutely no fashion opposed to itself. So,
while Contradictory Christology, as I advance it, is not tied specifically to the Catholic church,
there's nothing in the great tradition of Catholic reliance on both faith and reason that demands
a commitment to the mainstream view of logic.

The Contradictory Christ. Jc Beall, Oxford University Press (2021). © Jc Beall.
DOI: 10.1093/oso/9780198852360.003.0002

should be shaken. A better-founded account of logical consequence, one that preserves the mainstream account as a special case (i.e., a proper super-relation), is available.

This chapter provides an account of logical consequence and its relation to true theories, with special attention to the space of possibilities that logical consequence, as an entailment relation, recognizes – that is, the space of 'logical possibilities' – and the many (usually proper) sub-spaces of logical possibilities utilized by our true theories. The chapter advances a so-called subclassical account of logical consequence, an account that involves a wider space of logical possibilities than the narrow space involved in the mainstream account of logic. My aim throughout is to present just the bare minimum, keeping the ideas at a big-picture level while providing enough precision to convey key results.[2]

2.1 Entailment relations in general

Systematic theories are governed by so-called consequence relations (much more on which below). Consequence relations, for present purposes, are *entailment relations*. Logic (-al consequence) itself is a special such entailment relation; it's the focus of this chapter. Before turning to logical consequence more specifically, it's useful to review a few basic ideas about entailment relations. As entailment relations are relations on languages, rehearsal of the former requires rehearsal of the latter, and so I briefly rehearse, in a very big-picture way, the ideas of languages that are relevant to (a big-picture discussion of) entailment relations. Of course, 'real languages' – so-called natural languages in the wild (so to speak) – are wildly complicated and ever-growing beasts. Languages are fascinating in reality, too fascinating to talk about in any detail. For present purposes, I focus only on a simple but very standard model (or picture) of languages useful for reviewing the relevant idea of entailment relations.[3]

2.1.1 Very big picture

Entailment relations are (so-called binary) relations in (or, as logicians often say, on) languages, relating a sentence or a set of sentences to another

---

[2] Except for a few additions and clarifications, this chapter overlaps with Beall 2019*a*.
[3] And even here my sketch is highly selective in the features of languages discussed.

sentence. The sentence to which some sentence (or set of sentences) is related is said to be *entailed* by (or, as below, a consequence of) the sentence or set of sentences. And this relation is one of 'necessity' in the sense that it holds if and only if there's no possibility of a counterexample, no possibility in which the would-be entailing sentence (or set of sentences) is true but the would-be entailed sentence – the would-be consequence – is untrue.

There are a few central pieces in a picture of entailment: a language, a space (or set or class or etc.) of possibilities, and relations of truth and falsity between sentences of the language and the given possibilities. I quickly review the relevant ideas of a 'language' and the idea of true-at-possibility and false-at-possibility relations below. But the gist is available in a basic picture.

Think of a big space – or set or class or universe – of possibilities. Whatever else these possibilities are, they come equipped with a set of objects (viz., the objects that exist at the possibility) and properties and relations of such objects. (These 'properties' and 'relations' are modeled as nothing more nor less than sets of the objects, sets of ordered pairs of such objects for binary relations, and so on.) Now, every language, for present purposes, comes equipped with a set of sentences. The 'meaning' of such sentences supplies the conditions necessary and sufficient for a sentence's being true at a possibility or false at a possibility: knowing the meaning of a sentence is knowing the conditions under which the sentence is true and the conditions under which the sentence is false.[4] Now, returning to the big space of possibilities, each point is related to all sentences of the language by *true-at* and *false-at* relations. Take any sentence A in the language, and any possibility x in the big space, and there's an answer on whether x 'makes true' the sentence A and whether x 'makes false' the sentence A. Stepping back, you can look at the full space of possibilities and see whether, for example, a sentence is true at all of them, false at all of them, true (respectively, false) at none of them, or true (respectively, false) at a proper some of them. But you needn't restrict your sights only to sentences one-by-one; you can consider pairs of sentences in a given order, for example, you can consider the sentences A and B in that order (or in the converse direction). Here, going in the A-to-B direction, you can see whether there's a possibility in which A is true but B is untrue (i.e., A stands in the true-at relation to the given possibility, but B does not stand in the true-at relation to the given possibility). If there is

---

[4] I am not hereby endorsing this familiar picture as the full truth about meaning, although it is probably true as a partial account. Lewis (1975) gives a classic discussion of different accounts of linguistic (and in particular sentential) meaning.

such a point, we call it a *counterexample* to the would-be entailment from A to B. And, of course, you don't need to restrict your sights only to sentence-sentence pairs; you can likewise evaluate set-sentence pairs, where the set contains sentences from the given language. In this case, a counterexample to the would-be entailment claim from the set X of sentences to sentence B is some point (i.e., possibility) in the space at which *all* sentences in X are true (i.e., stand in the true-at relation to the given point) but B untrue (i.e., B doesn't stand in the true-at relation to the given point).

And now we have at least the big-picture sketch of entailment. In particular, an entailment relation on a language is an absence-of-counterexample relation between sentences (or sets thereof) of the language and sentences of the language. The counterexamples are possibilities in some space of possibilities over which the meanings of the sentences – enough to determine true-at and false-at relations for all such sentences at all such points – are defined.

That's the big picture, and that's roughly enough to get a rough sense of *logical* entailment – the key focus of this chapter. Still, even if mildly redundant, so as to get a slightly finer sense of some of the bigger points, it's useful to walk through a rough and ready review of the relevant idea of 'languages', just enough to make the target discussion of logical consequence (i.e., logical entailment) an easy segue.

2.1.2 Languages and their salient parts

Languages, for present purposes, have a 'syntax' and 'semantics'. The syntax specifies the various bits of the language to which meanings (semantics) are attached. For present purposes, only the barest of bits are relevant.

2.1.2.1 Alphabet and other bits
The alphabet, including so-called punctuation, is whatever is used to give the language its physical – or, generally, its distinguishing or identifying – shape or form, so to speak. 'B' and 'b' are alphabetical items of English, as are ')' and '(' and '!' and so on, at least on the relevant sense of 'alphabet', which is basically the clothing or medium or fabric or whathaveyou out of which the language's sentences are packaged.

2.1.2.2 Singular terms
Singular terms in English are items such as 'Christ', 'The Dome', 'the set of all cats', '2' and so on. Syntactically, without invoking their intended meaning

or semantic role, the singular terms are just whatever the official syntax (or grammar) lists as singular terms.

Important simplification: because the chief issues of this chapter allow as much, I assume that the singular terms of the languages that, for present purposes, illustrate entailment relations are one and all names – not definite (let alone indefinite) descriptions, demonstratives, or the like, even though such items are generally classified as singular terms in English and other natural languages.

2.1.2.3 Predicates

Predicates in English are items such as 'is a koala', 'is standing behind', 'is between . . . and . . . ', and so on. Syntactically, without invoking their intended semantic role, predicates can be defined in terms of what they do to make 'sentences' (another bit of language defined below). For present purposes, a *predicate* is an item that, when combined with the right number of singular terms, results in a sentence (of the given language). The *right number of singular terms* is determined by the 'arity' or degree of the predicate: a *unary* predicate takes exactly one singular term to make a sentence; a *binary* predicate takes exactly two singular terms to make a sentence; and so on. A predicate is called an *n-ary predicate* if and only if n is the arity of the predicate.

Important simplification: the 'slots' of a predicate. For ease of exposition, I assume that each n-ary predicate of a language comes with exactly n many 'slots', where these (usually invisible) slots are the only places into which singular terms can be plugged to make sentences of the language. (In English, 'is standing' is a unary predicate whose slot is at the front: 'Max is standing' is the result of plugging the singular term 'Max' into the unique slot of the given predicate, while 'Agnes is standing between Max and Virgil' is the result of plugging 'Agnes', 'Max' and 'Virgil' – in that order – into the three slots of the given ternary predicate. And so on.)

2.1.2.4 Sentences: atomic

Sentences in English are items such as 'Christ is a contradictory being', 'Tractors are useful tools', 'Max is a koala', 'Agnes is smarter than both Max and Bentley', and so on. Syntactically, without invoking meaning, a language's sentences are whatever the syntax (or grammar) declares them to be. The key job of a syntax is to define the language's set of sentences.

For present purposes we focus – just in this run through relevant ideas of a language – on the simplest sort of sentences, namely, so-called *atomic sentences*. These are defined in terms of the first two syntactic categories:

- An *atomic sentence* (of a given language) is the result of plugging exactly n many singular terms (from the language) into the slots of any n-ary predicate.

Hence, in English, 'Agnes is a koala' is a sentence, since 'Agnes' is a singular term (indeed, a name) and 'is a koala' is a unary predicate with its unique slot at the front, right where 'Agnes' sits in 'Agnes is a koala'.

2.1.3 Meanings: denotation, true-of and false-of relations

The syntactic bits and bobs are necessary but insufficient ingredients of a language. Indeed, unless one is supremely keenly into the mere syntactic mechanisms of logical systems, the driving stuff of a language involves meaning – the semantic bits and bobs of a language.

As with real syntax, the real semantics of a real (i.e., natural) language is really difficult. Present purposes do not demand any of the difficulties. All that's needed for present purposes is enough meaning to review *entailment relations* on a language. And this is largely achieved via (models of) truth and falsity conditions, conditions built out of a few fundamental semantic relations.

Just as the central syntactic bits of a language (viz., in our example, the atomic sentences) are built from a few primitive parts (viz., singular terms and predicates), so too with the central semantic bits.

2.1.3.1 Singular terms: denotation

The fundamental semantical relation is a so-called mapping relation between singular terms (names, for present purposes) and objects. The relation is standardly called *denotation*, and the object to which a term (name) is related is often called the *referent* or simply *denotation* of the given term. In English, 'Christ' denotes Christ; 'Max' denotes Max; 'Agnes' denotes Agnes; and so on.

The meaning of a singular term (name), for present purposes, is simply whatever the language's denotation function specifies as its referent.[5] In short, the meaning of a name (singular term) is its denotation or referent.

---

[5] In the philosophy of language, this is called an *extensional* account of the meaning. For present purposes, I simply 'go extensional' for the meanings of all sub-sentential expressions (including predicates), as further complications – such as the 'intension' (i.e., the unchanging meaning that determines the 'extensional meaning') – are unnecessary for present purposes.

2.1.3.2 Predicates: true-of and false-of

The other two fundamental semantical relations are the *true-of* and *false-of* relations between predicates and objects. These relations relate unary predicates to individual objects (one at a time); they relate binary predicates to pairs of such objects (in a given order); they relate ternary predicates to triples of objects (in a given order); and so on. For present purposes, I focus only on unary predicates, just for simplicity. When a unary predicate is true-of (false-of) an object, the object is said to be in the *extension* (respectively, *antiextension*) of the predicate, where, in turn, the extension of a predicate is the set containing all objects of which the predicate is true (i.e., all objects to which the true-of relation relates the predicate), and the antiextension the set of objects of which the predicate is false (i.e., all objects to which the false-of relation relates the predicate).

The meaning of a predicate, for present purposes, is simply the pair of sets assigned to it by the true-of and false-of relations, namely, the pair consisting of the predicate's given extension and the predicate's given antiextension.

2.1.4 Meanings of (atomic) sentences: truth and falsity conditions

With the true-of and false-of relations, together with denotation, a language's (atomic) sentences achieve their meanings by way of a familiar recipe two lines of which are very familiar:

- An atomic sentence is *true* if and only if the denotation of the singular term (e.g., name) is in the extension of the predicate.
- An atomic sentence is *false* if and only if the denotation of the singular term (e.g., name) is in the antiextension of the predicate.

This account of truth and falsity conditions for simple (atomic) sentences should appear to be nearly obvious, perhaps even needless to say. Truth and falsity conditions, when explicitly given, are generally obvious, at least for atomic sentences, since they specify nothing more nor less than the in-effect primitive base case: a subject-predicate sentence is true (respectively, false) if and only if the given predicate is true of (respectively, false of) the given subject. From English:

- *Example from English:* 'Agnes is reading' is true if and only if the denotation of 'Agnes' (viz., Agnes) is in the set of objects of which 'is reading' is true.
- *Example from English:* 'Agnes is reading' is false if and only if the denotation of 'Agnes' (viz., Agnes) is in the set of objects of which 'is reading' is false.

And that's basically it, except for one critical generalization that may appear at first to be slightly complicated.

The simplicity of truth and falsity conditions for atomic sentences is as above, but – and here is the slight complication – there is more to truth and falsity conditions *as meanings of sentences* than merely specifying the actual conditions under which sentences are true and false. What's involved is the 'full slate' of possible conditions under which sentences are true (respectively, false): to give the meaning of a sentence is to specify not only the actual conditions under which the sentence is true (respectively, false); one must specify *all possible conditions* under which – or *at which* (or *in which*) – the sentences are true (respectively, false).

One might ask: what is the nature of such 'possible conditions' or, more generally, of such 'possibilities'? That question is not for this book.[6] A common practice, at least for semantics, is to sidestep the question of what such possibilities ultimately are, and instead give 'truth and falsity conditions' in terms of *models* of possibilities, where these come equipped with a 'domain of objects' (a set of objects that models the set of existing objects at some possibility) and properties and relations on the domain – namely, sets of objects from the domain, sets of pairs of such objects, sets of triples of such objects, and so on, where these sets model the relevant properties and relations, or at least the relevant extensions and antiextensions. This practice suffices for present purposes.

The key semantical relations in all of this are the true-at (or true-in) and false-at (or false-in) relations. These central semantic relations are defined, in the basic (atomic) case, in terms of the other key relations: an atomic sentence is *true-in-a-possibility (model)* if and only if the given denotation in that possibility (model) is in the given extension in that possibility (model); an atomic sentence is *false-in-a-possibility (model)* if and only if the given

---

[6] Discussion of that question is available in many (many) works. A classic is by Lewis (1986). An elementary step into surrounding issues is by Rea (2014).

denotation in that possibility (model) is in the given antiextension in that possibility (model). And that's basically it.

The key idea is that the meaning of a sentence gives you everything you need to evaluate the sentence for truth or falsity at any relevant possibility. Every possibility is one at which a meaningful sentence can be evaluated with respect to the truth-at and false-at relations (in effect, evaluated with respect to truth and falsity). And this brings us full circle to entailment.

2.1.5 Entailment relations on a language

Entailment relations naturally fall out of the foregoing ideas.[7] Every language has entailment relations on it. Why? Answer: every language has meaningful sentences; the meanings determine true-at and false-at relations at possibilities; and entailment relations are simply absence-of-counterexample relations over spaces of possibilities and the sentences of a language. Consider, by way of example, the following English claim:

1. That Agnes is a living feline animal entails that Agnes has a functioning heart inside her body.

This entailment claim is refuted by counterexamples – relevant possibilities – in which Agnes is living but is living only via external contraptions that circulate blood through Agnes' circulatory system.

Entailment relations can differ from one another depending on the vocabulary to which they are tied. In philosophy and theology, vocabulary such as 'God', 'good', 'it is necessary that', and so on are central pieces of the target languages over which key entailment relations are defined.

Logical entailment – or, as below, 'logic' (for short) – is a special entailment relation; it's keyed to so-called logical vocabulary. The relation of logical entailment (logical consequence) is the central focus of the rest of this chapter.

---

[7] And the following ideas should now begin to feel slightly redundant (or more redundant, as the case may be), but this should facilitate the segue into the focus on logical entailment.

2.2 The role of logic in general and in theology

Logic is the common foundation of all (so-called closed) theories; it's part of the (extra-logical, stronger) 'consequence' or 'entailment' relation for our true theories. These ideas can be spelled out with reference to logic's role in theology.

2.2.1 Theology and consequence

Christian theology is a theory of God, just as macro physics is a theory of the macro-physical world and just as mathematical theories are theories of their respective mathematical phenomena (numbers, categories, sets, whathaveyou).[8] When we construct our theology (our theory of God) we begin by adding truths of God, including (for example) that God is triune, that Christ has two (complementary) natures, that God is omniscient, and so on for whatever we, as theologians (as theorists of God), take to be true of God – including, of course, truths about what God is not, what is false of God (e.g., that it is false that God is limited, false that God is evil, etc.).[9]

When theorists aim to construct a true theory, they aim to construct as complete a theory as possible. In particular, the resulting theory should not only contain the initial thrown-in truths (e.g., that God is triune, that Christ has two natures, etc.); the theory should also contain *whatever follows from the truths in the theory*; it should contain all of the *consequences* of the theory's claims. The question is: what is meant by 'follows from' and 'consequences' in this context?

This is where consequence relations enter. A consequence relation for a set of claims is an entailment relation.[10] In particular, a consequence relation tells you *what claims follow*, according to that relation, from your given set of

---

[8] My use of 'theology' to in-effect conveniently abbreviate 'theological theory' is not intended to suggest that the practice of theology – 'doing theology' – involves nothing beyond theory construction. Still, as a truth-seeking discipline, theology aims at the true theory of God, and the resulting true theory is called '(the) true theology' in the same way that the true theory of physical reality is called '(the) true physics'. For recent discussion of various contemporary conceptions of systematic theology, see Torrance 2019.

[9] The *source* of our knowledge of theological truth is an issue for epistemology; my topic in this book concerns only the record – the theory – of our true theology, not its source.

[10] In more detail: I assume that target consequence relations are what are classified as 'closure relations' along the lines initially explored by Tarski (1956). This imposes certain technical constraints on what counts as a consequence relation; but for my purposes I leave the details aside. (Everything I say is compatible with the requisite conditions on closure relations.)

claims, where 'follows from' is understood as entailment – as necessary truth preservation over some target space of possibilities.

Example: consider the theory of knowledge. That theory contains the following truth:

2. It is known that 1+1=2.

And there are many other thrown-in truths of that form: *it is known that p* where *p* is some known truth. But there are many 'it is known that...'-free claims in our true theory of knowledge too. An example:

3. 1+1=2.

Why is (3) in our true – and as-complete-as-possible – theory of knowledge? Answer: because (3) is a *consequence* of (2), and (2) is in our theory of knowledge. Our best theory of knowledge has a consequence relation according to which, for any sentence *p* in the language, *p* follows from – is entailed by, is a consequence of – the claim *it is known that p*.

There is nothing special about the theory of knowledge. The construction of true theories involves the construction of consequence (closure) relations for those theories – an entailment relation that serves to 'complete' the theory (as far as possible) by churning out all of the truths that follow from (that are entailed by) the claims in the theory. Our true theory of (for example) temporal phenomena has it that *it is false that p* follows from *it is always true that it is false that p*; our true theory of (for example) metaphysical possibility has it that *it is metaphysically possible that p* follows from *it is true that p*.

Such theory-specific consequence relations are just that: theory-specific. The consequence relation governing knowledge claims (i.e., claims of the form *it is known that...*) is not involved in the consequence relation governing the theory of arithmetic (unless the theory is also in part about explicit knowledge of arithmetic). The theorist's task is to construct a set of truths about a target phenomenon and close that set of truths under the consequence relation that, by the theorist's lights, is the right relation to 'complete' the true theory of the given phenomenon.

And theology is no different. Theologians must not only add various basic truths about God but also 'complete' (as far as possible) the theory via a consequence relation. According to the consequence relation of true christian theology, *that it is false that p* follows from any sentence *p* that claims the existence of a rival god or, for that matter, any sentence *p* that limits God's powers or authority. While theologians have not always been explicit about their target consequence relation they have nonetheless assumed one in their systematic pursuit of the 'complete' (as possible) truth of God – the true theology.

Without a consequence (closure) relation our theories remain inadequate; they fail to contain truths that are entailed by the given set of truths. Inasmuch as theorists, and theologians in particular, aim to give as complete a theory of the target phenomenon as possible, the reliance on a consequence relation for our theory is required.

But what have such theory-specific consequence relations to do with logic's role in theories?

2.2.2 Consequence and (formal) logical consequence

Logic is a very special consequence (entailment, closure) relation. Logic is the common core of all (closed) theories;[11] it is at the bottom of all of the (extra-logical, theory-specific) consequence relations of our true theories. While the theory-specific consequence relation for our theory of knowledge is different from the consequence relation for our theory of arithmetic (or necessity, or God) the two consequence relations share a common elementary core: namely, logic. Logic itself does not say anything peculiar about knowledge claims, arithmetical claims, modal claims or theological claims; logic ignores the specific subject matter of those sorts of claims (be it knowledge, arithmetic, modality, or God) and treats them as it treats claims about any subject matter whatsoever. In this way, logic is said to be 'universal' and 'topic-neutral'.

Logic's universality and foundational role in all of our true (closed) theories is achieved by logic's narrow focus: it focuses only on so-called logical vocabulary. Chief examples of logical vocabulary (and, for purposes of this chapter, the only canvassed examples) are the so-called boolean quartet:[12]

---

[11] For present purposes (skipping technical details), think of a closed theory as a set of claims closed under a consequence relation such that (among other things) if a sentence is a consequence of something in the theory then that sentence is in the theory.

[12] This is an incomplete list of logical vocabulary. The logical vocabulary extends beyond the list below to the standard first-order vocabulary involving logical quantifiers (though not, on my view, an identity predicate). Again, for present purposes it suffices to focus on the following basic vocabulary.

- Truth (or null) operator: *it is true that . . .*
- Falsity (or negation) operator: *it is false that . . .*
- Conjunction: *. . . and . . .*
- Disjunction: *either . . . or . . . (or both)*

Logical consequence – logical entailment – is a so-called *formal* relation: it looks only at certain 'forms' of sentences, namely, the ones individuated in terms of logical vocabulary. In particular, logic recognizes only a limited list of forms:

- *Atomic sentences*: any sentence which is *free* of logical vocabulary.[13]
- *Nullations (truth claims)*: any sentence of the form *it is true that . . . .*[14]
- *Negations (falsity claims)*: any sentence of the form *it is false that . . . .*
- *Conjunctions*: any sentence of the given (logical-conjunction) form, namely, *. . . and . . .* where 'and' is logical conjunction.
- *Disjunctions*: any sentence of the given (logical-disjunction) form, namely, *. . . or . . .* where 'or' is logical disjunction.

Logic recognizes only the foregoing kinds (forms) of sentences, and it classifies entailments only in terms of the limited list of forms. Important to note is that logic treats all atomic claims on par: logic itself sees no difference *in logically relevant content* between 'God is good' and 'Hogwarts is fictional'; such a difference – and the resulting difference in entailments – arises only in extra-logical, theory-specific consequence relations.

Examples of common logical entailments are the following, where $\wedge$ is logical conjunction, $\vee$ logical disjunction, $\neg$ the falsity (or negation) operator, $\dagger$ the truth (or null) operator, and p and q are any (declarative) sentences:

- p logically entails $p \vee q$.
- $p \wedge q$ logically entails q (and also p).
- $\neg p \wedge \neg q$ is a logical consequence of $\neg(p \vee q)$ (and vice versa).
- $\neg p \vee \neg q$ is a logical consequence of $\neg(p \wedge q)$ (and vice versa).
- p logically entails $\dagger p$ (and vice versa).
- $\neg\neg p$ logically entails $\dagger p$ (and vice versa).

---

[13] Throughout, 'sentence' shall be used to pick out *declarative* sentences – sentences that declare something about (versus asking or commanding something of) reality.

[14] This category is often ignored, since logic treats its truth operator as (logically) redundant. In much of what follows I follow suit by ignoring, for the most part, the truth operator.

Logic is formal in that its consequence relation holds only in virtue of the given logical forms. For example, anything of the form $\neg p \wedge \neg q$ logically entails anything of the form $\neg(p \vee q)$. And logic says nothing about any 'forms' that go beyond its recognized list.

Logical entailment, like any entailment relation, is a relation of necessary truth preservation over relevant possibilities – in this case, the so-called logical possibilities (i.e., the possibilities recognized by logic). The recipe for logical entailment is absence of counterexample:

> L. Let X be a set of sentences, and p any sentence. Then X logically entails p (i.e., p is a logical consequence of X) if and only if there is no possibility in which everything in X is true but p is untrue. (A counterexample is a possibility in which everything in X is true but p untrue.)

Here, 'possibility' picks out whatever logic recognizes as possible. While there is ongoing debate about which possibilities are logical possibilities (i.e., recognized by logic's entailment relation) one matter is settled: logic plays its universal, foundational role in our theories by recognizing the widest space of possibilities. In physical theory, the space of possibilities is restricted to those (logical) possibilities that obey physical laws. In arithmetic the space of possibilities is restricted to those (logical) possibilities that obey the laws of arithmetic. In theology the space of possibilities is restricted to those (logical) possibilities that obey the truths about God.

Logic is the common core of all theory-specific consequence relations in virtue of logic's recognizing the widest space of possibilities. The possibilities in terms of which a theory-specific entailment relation is defined (i.e., in terms of which the theory's class of would-be counterexamples is defined) are one and all logical possibilities. The theory-specific consequence relations restrict the space of logical possibilities in order to focus on target, phenomenon-specific entailments (i.e., entailments that aren't recognized by all consequence relations for true theories); but they do not reject or otherwise transgress logical entailments.

In the end, logic's role in theology is its role in all of our true and 'complete' (as possible) theories: namely, to deliver the logical consequences of the claims in our theories. Logic is involved in all consequence relations for our true theories, including our theory of God (i.e., our theology). Logic achieves this universal role – the foundation of all entailment (or closure) relations on our true theories – in virtue of recognizing the widest space of possibilities. It's not that 'anything goes' by logic's lights; but a vast array of otherwise very strange possibilities is recognized by logic.

2.2.3 Logic and standard logic

At least since Aquinas, whose work reflected (one reading of) Aristotle, the range of logical possibilities has standardly been thought to be narrower than I, along with other so-called subclassical-logic theorists, take it to be. The standard class of possibilities is modeled by so-called classical-logic models. The term 'classical' does not denote Aristotle's logic, since Aristotle's logic was both impoverished (lacking, e.g., adequate quantificational resources and much else) and also arguably at odds with so-called classical logic (Priest, 1998). In fact, what is today called 'classical logic' is a fairly recent construction ushered in largely by the philosophers Boole, Peirce, Ladd-Franklin, Frege, Russell, and Whitehead.

This book is not the place to rehearse the history of logic or the many debates on whether the standard account of logic gets things right. By my lights, for reasons argued elsewhere (Beall, 2009; Belnap, 1977; Dunn, 1966, 1976; Priest, 2006; Priest *et al.*, 2004; Routley, 1979; Routley and Meyer, 1976), the correct account of logic is in fact weaker than the standard one: the space of logical possibilities is much wider than the standard account takes it to be; the set of logically valid entailments (or 'logically valid forms') is smaller than the standard set. For present purposes my aim in this chapter is only to present the weaker account (one that I believe to be the right account), leaving debate for other venues.

2.3 Logic: subclassical

The aim of this section (and its subsections) is to present, as concisely as possible (without obliterating user-friendliness), the target account of logic: namely, what is called 'first-degree entailment' (FDE), an account applied on a wide range of philosophical fronts by many philosophers but most famously explored by Anderson and Belnap (1975); Anderson *et al.* (1992); Dunn (1966, 1976). I believe but, for present purposes, shall only assume that FDE is the correct account of logic (qua universal consequence relation in the sense given above).[15] While arguing for the truth of this assumption is too much for this book, I shall defend the claim in some of the objections and replies (see §4).

2.3.1 Formal language

As above (see §2.2.2), logical consequence is a *formal* entailment relation; it holds in virtue of 'logical form'. The target forms are specified by logical vocabulary. Because the main action of the present chapter can be seen at the so-called propositional (or sentential) level, we restrict the following to just that level – indeed, restricting to just the so-called monadic predicates for simplicity.[16]

Following standard practice we use models – and an artificial, formal 'model language' – to specify the target entailment relation. Entailment, as above, is necessary truth-preservation over a space of relevant possibilities. In logic these possibilities are modeled by some sort of mathematical structure (sets, functions, relations); and the idea of a sentence's being true (false) at a possibility is modeled by relations that are defined on the given structures. Despite the level of mathematical abstraction the target remains always on 'real logical consequence' for our 'real language'. The 'logically valid forms' that are generated by the mathematical account are advanced as the 'real' logically valid forms.

In what follows the syntax (grammar, vocabulary, and definition of sentences) is presented first, followed by the semantics (model of truth and falsity conditions for the sentences), followed by the central target: namely, the logical consequence relation (logic).

2.3.1.1 Syntax
The basic alphabet (vocabulary) of the language are as follows.

1. Vocabulary:
   (a) Logical expressions:
       i. Unary connectives: † and ¬
       ii. Binary connectives: ∧ and ∨

---

[15] For arguments towards this conclusion see Beall 2017.

[16] A generalization to the full stock of (standard) first-order vocabulary is not difficult but, again, is not necessary for purposes of this chapter. (The presentation here involves monadic predicates – versus the even simpler 'sentential variables' – to give at least some sense of how atomic sentences are modeled as both true and false.)

(b) Extralogical expressions:
    i. Unary predicates: 'P', 'Q', 'R' with or without numerical subscripts (unary: they take one name to make a sentence)
    ii. Names: lowercase letters of English, with or without numerical subscripts
(c) Alogical expressions:
    i. Punctuation: left and right parentheses (viz., ')' and '(').

The syntax, while on its own (apart from a semantics) meaningless, is motivated by our target logic. In particular, the unary connectives ('unary' because they take exactly one sentence to make a sentence) will be treated in the semantics as logic's truth and falsity operators, and the binary connectives will be treated as the logical conjunction and disjunction operators.

Worth noting is that the predicates and names in the class of extralogical expressions are not necessary for specifying the logic; they are in there to add (I hope) some illumination on how atomic sentences are formally interpreted (see semantics below). One can simplify the syntax by ignoring any structure in atomic sentences and simply having standard 'propositional letters' as atomic sentences.

The *sentences* of the language are defined as follows.

2. Sentences of the language:
    (a) Atomics: let G be a predicate and η a name. Then G followed by η (viz., '$G\eta$') is an atomic sentence.
    (b) Molecular (Compound): If A and B are sentences of the language, then so too are $\dagger A$, $\neg A$, $(A \wedge B)$ and $(A \vee B)$.
    (c) Nothing else is a sentence of the language (except what follows from the first two clauses).

Examples of atomic sentences are Pa, Rb_{22}, and Qd. (See the list of predicates and the list of names under vocabulary, and then consult the definition of atomics above.) Examples of molecular sentences (i.e., sentences that contain at least one logical expression) are $\dagger Pa$, $(\neg Rb_{22} \vee (Qd \wedge Pa))$, and $(Qd \vee Pa)$.[17]

---

[17] To see that these are in fact official sentences, consult the definition of sentences above and simply let A be Qd, B be Pa, in which case, for example, $(Qd \wedge Pa)$ counts as a sentence; and now let A be Rb_{22}, in which case, $\neg Rb_{22}$ counts as a sentence; and now let A be $\neg Rb_{22}$ and B be $(Qd \wedge Pa)$, in which case $(\neg Rb_{22} \vee (Qd \wedge Pa))$ counts as a sentence.

2.3.1.2 Semantics: towards truth and falsity conditions

The aim, again, is to precisely specify the logical consequence relation, which is an entailment relation, which is a truth-preserving relation over relevant possibilities. To specify the target truth-preserving relation for our model language we need to have an account of truth and falsity conditions for the sentences of the language.

As in standard accounts of logic a sentence's having a truth value (or, generally, 'semantic status') boils down to what's happening at the atomic level. In other words, our logical connectives are all 'truth-functional' in a familiar way: the semantic value of a sentence is a function of the semantic values of the atomic sentences. In this way, the semantic action takes place at the atomic level.

Atomic sentences get to have a semantic value (be it truth, falsity or something else) in a familiar way. Examples: if the subject term of the sentence picks out (denotes) an object of which the predicate term is true, then the given sentence is (at least) true; if the subject term of the sentence picks out an object of which the predicate term is false, then the given atomic sentence is (at least) false.[18] So, atomic sentences get their values in terms of what their parts (in our simple language, a unary predicate and a name) denote.

In general, think of the 'possibilities' involved in logic as modeled by certain mathematical models. For our purposes, models contain both a denotation function δ, which supplies a semantic value to predicates and names, and a domain D of objects – namely, all of the objects that exist according to the model.

2.3.1.3 Atomic sentences

A predicate G's semantic value is modeled as a pair $\langle G^+, G^- \rangle$, where G^+ (the so-called extension) contains all of the objects of which the predicate G is true, and G^- (the so-called antiextension) contains all of the objects of which G is false. Where δ is a denotation function for a model, the predicate G is given the semantic value $\delta(G) = \langle G^+, G^- \rangle$ in a model, while each name η is given a denotation $\delta(\eta)$ from the set D of objects in the model. These resources are then used to provide a semantic status for atomic sentences.

Truth and falsity conditions for atomic sentences are as follows, where δ is the 'denotation function' of a given model:

---

[18] The 'at least' is redundant in standard (so-called classical) accounts of logic; but it is not redundant in the account advanced here, namely, FDE. This will be clear below.

- *Truth in a model*: Atomic $G\eta$ is true-in-a-model iff $\delta(\eta)$ is in G^+.
- *Falsity in a model*: Atomic $G\eta$ is false-in-a-model iff $\delta(\eta)$ is in G^-.

Of paramount importance is the question of what constraints logic imposes on the interpretation of predicates (i.e., on the denotation of predicates). The issue may be seen by considering two salient constraints.

- *Exhaustion*: every model is 'exhaustive' with respect to every predicate in the sense that *every object in the domain* is either in G^+ or in G^-.[19]
- *Exclusion*: every model is 'exclusive' with respect to every predicate in the sense that *no object in the domain* is in both G^+ and G^-.[20]

On the so-called classical account, logic imposes both exhaustion and exclusion. Logic, on that account, is exhaustive: it recognizes no possibility in which an object fails to be in either the extension or antiextension of a predicate – no possibility in which a predicate fails to be either at least true of the object or at least false of the object. (This rules out the logical possibility of 'truth-value gaps', where a sentence is neither true nor false for some reason – a sort of indeterminacy of semantic value.) Moreover, logic, on the 'classical' account, is exclusive: it recognizes no possibility in which an object falls into both the extension and antiextension of a predicate – no possibility in which a predicate is both true and false of an object. (This rules out the logical possibility of 'truth-value gluts', where a sentence is both true and false for some reason – a sort of overdeterminacy of semantic value.)

These constraints are overly strict from an alternative (viz., FDE) account of logic. The issue is too complex to argue here, but at least one consideration can be advanced. In particular, the classical-logic constraints (above) are very, very well-motivated when one focuses one's attention on a standard diet of examples from sciences like mathematics – the very diet to which the classical-logic account was historically directed. But reality is more than just mathematics. Reality appears to contain some surprising (however rare) phenomena that don't naturally fit into the confines of classical-logic assumptions. Reflection on language's strange phenomena (e.g., vagueness, paradoxical phenomena, and more) don't obviously fall into the confines of (classical-logic-governed) mathematics. Moreover, and most pressing for present purposes, reality involves a theological realm and its complex

---

[19] In set-theoretic notation: $G^+ \cup G^- = D$ where D is the domain of the model.
[20] In set-theoretic notation: $G^+ \cap G^- = \emptyset$ where $\emptyset$ is the empty set.

phenomena – including, from orthodox christian theology, the fundamental problem of christology. It may well be that all such extra-mathematical phenomena are truly described by a classical-logic-like consequence relation; but there is no obvious reason to think that logic itself demands as much.

Logic, on the FDE account, imposes *neither* exhaustion nor exclusion on its predicates. A model – representing one of the possibilities that logic recognizes – *may* treat a predicate as exclusive; it may treat it as exhaustive; it may treat it as both. But on the FDE account there are also models in which a predicate may be neither true nor false of an object – the resulting atomic sentence 'gappy' in the model – and there are models in which a predicate may be both true and false (a 'glutty' model).

What the FDE account does *not* do is reject any classical-logic models. The account accepts all classical-logic models as genuine models (as representations of possibilities that logic recognizes); the account simply *expands* the space of models to recognize ones that go beyond the narrow confines of the classical-logic space. What this means is that if there is a classical-logic counterexample to an argument, then there is an FDE counterexample too – since FDE's space of models includes the narrower classical-logic ones. But the converse fails: FDE recognizes more possibilities (more genuine models) than the classical-logic perspective allows, and so recognizes more candidate counterexamples than classical logic recognizes.

2.3.1.4   Semantic values for molecular sentences

Atomic sentences achieve their semantic values – or semantic statuses – as above (see §2.3.1.3). Models are likewise as above, with no constraint that requires exhaustion or exclusion on predicates. This gives four possibilities for an atomic sentence:

- Just-true: the denoted subject (i.e., denotation of the name) is in the extension of the given predicate but not in the antiextension.
- Just-false: the denoted subject is in the antiextension of the given predicate but not in the extension.
- Gap (gappy): the denoted subject is in neither the extension nor the antiextension.
- Glut (glutty): the denoted subject is in both the extension and the antiextension.

Following terminology from Belnap (1977) we shall say that an atomic sentence is *at least true (false)* iff the denoted subject is at least in the extension (at least in the antiextension) of the given predicate. Then truth and falsity conditions for molecular sentences are as follows, where A and B are any sentences:[21]

- Nullations: $\dagger A$ is at least true in model m iff A is at least true in model m.
- Nullations: $\dagger A$ is at least false in model m iff A is at least false in model m.
- Negations: $\neg A$ is at least true in model m iff A is at least false in model m.
- Negations: $\neg A$ is at least false in model m iff A is at least true in model m.
- Disjunctions: $A \vee B$ is at least true in model m iff either A is at least true in m or B is at least true in m.
- Disjunctions: $A \vee B$ is at least false in model m iff both A is at least false in m and B is at least false in m.
- Conjunctions: $A \wedge B$ is at least true in model m iff both A is at least true in m and B is at least true in m.
- Conjunctions: $A \wedge B$ is at least false in model m iff either A is at least false in m or B is at least false in m.

What is important to emphasize, as discussed again below, is that these truth and falsity conditions *are precisely the same conditions* used in the standard classical-logic account. The difference is that the classical-logic account ignores the logical possibilities of gaps and gluts, and so both the 'at least' phrase and the falsity conditions are redundant in the classical-logic picture. But, again, if one's aim is to accommodate the full space of logical possibilities – and not just those that are relevant to (for example) standard mathematics – then the fuller account of truth and falsity conditions is required.

2.4 Logic: the target consequence relation

Finally, the target relation – namely, logical consequence – may be specified in terms of the given FDE models and the given true-at and false-at conditions. The consequence relation is a relation between a set of sentences X and a sentence A. The definition is as follows:

---

[21] Nullations are included here for completeness (and the symmetry of the boolean quartet) but shall be ignored – because redundant – in what follows.

- *X logically entails A* (equivalently: *A* is a *logical consequence* of *X*) iff there is no model in which everything in *X* is at least true but *A* is not even at least true.

When *X* logically entails *A* we say that the argument from *X* to *A* is *logically valid* – that is, valid by logic's lights. We use ⊢ to represent the logical consequence relation, sometimes writing '*X* ⊢ *A*' as shorthand for the claim that *X* logically entails *A* according to the given (FDE) consequence relation.[22]

2.5 Salient logical (in-) validities

Some key *invalid argument forms*, relevant to the project of any true contradictory christology (or, more generally, contradictory theology) are these, where '*X* ⊬ *A*' indicates that *X* does not logically entail *A*:

- *A* ∧ ¬*A* ⊬ *B*. (Hence, as far as logic is concerned, a theory can contain a contradiction *A*∧¬*A* without thereby entailing all sentences whatsoever.)
- *B* ⊬ *A* ∨ ¬*A*. (Hence, a theory is not required by logic alone to contain all instances of the so-called law of excluded middle – a principle that may well be in force for some important theory-specific consequence relations, but isn't required by logic itself.)

On the other hand, all standard De Morgan interaction between logical expressions remains in force as the chief concern of logic. For example, where ⊣⊢ indicates logical equivalence (i.e., two-way logical entailment):

- ¬(*A* ∧ *B*) ⊣⊢ ¬*A* ∨ ¬*B*.
- ¬(*A* ∨ *B*) ⊣⊢ ¬*A* ∧ ¬*B*.
- ¬¬*A* ⊣⊢ †*A* ⊣⊢ *A*.

In effect, the FDE picture is one in which logic demands De Morgan interaction among the logical expressions, but that is all that logic itself demands. The harder question of whether atomic sentences are 'gappy' or 'glutty' is

---

[22] When the set *X* contains exactly one sentence *B* we shall write '*B* ⊢ *A*' instead of the explicit {*B*} ⊢ *A*. Similarly, when the set *X* is empty we shall write '⊢ *A*' instead of the more explicit '∅ ⊢ *A*'. (This notation is not central for present purposes but is useful to have at hand.)

a theory-specific matter for the given phenomenon; logic itself recognizes possibilities in which atomic sentences take on any of the four (logically possible) semantic statuses.

2.6 Chief virtues of this account of logic

There are at least three salient virtues of this account of logic.

The first virtue is that the familiar truth and falsity conditions are maintained, as above. There is no revision of the truth or falsity conditions; there is instead a more complete and explicit account – and that's all. In this way the 'meanings' of the standard logical vocabulary remain as per the standard (classical-logic) account; it's just that the standard account is properly seen for what it has always been: namely, a restricted account. The standard account is a theory-specific consequence relation (e.g., for mathematical theories among others) that restricts its truth and falsity conditions only to the logical possibilities in which 'exclusion' and 'exhaustion' are satisfied. There is nothing at all wrong with the resulting consequence relation on such a restriction; it's just that, as above, the full space of logical possibilities demands a fuller and more explicit specification of truth and falsity conditions, namely, the ones involved in the given broader account.

A second virtue is that the resulting logic is clearly topic-neutral by not taking a stand on whether gappy or glutty atomic sentences are ruled out. Such an issue, as far as logic is concerned, is a topic-rich one for individual theories to figure out. While this is a virtue for an account of logic itself, it is a frustration for the epistemological process of determining the true theory of various phenomena; however, that's a different matter. Epistemology – or rational 'change in view' – is a complicated but distinct discipline from a theory of logical consequence (Beall, 2015; Harman, 1986).

A third virtue is most relevant to the principal project of a contradictory christology: namely, that logic does not force unique, strange phenomena into the cramped confines of classical-logic possibilities. While logic itself is silent on whether theorists *should* entertain a contradictory (glutty) theory of a given phenomenon – or, similarly, a gappy one, or an entirely 'classical-logic' theory – logic itself, contrary to the standard account, doesn't rule it out. And in the face of extraordinary or strikingly bizarre phenomena it is a good thing to have a very wide space of possibilities to work with in constructing a true theory of the rare entity.

3

Seven virtues

§1 answered the basic *what* question: what's the central claim of Contradictory Christology? §2 answered the pressing *how* question: how does the account avoid logical absurdity or logical incoherence? This chapter turns to the *why* question: Why accept Contradictory Christology over the many consistent accounts?

As the longstanding quest for a consistent account of Christ reveals, there are – to absolutely nobody's surprise – many, many, many abstract options for getting around the apparent contradiction of Christ. (And there are undoubtedly many more yet to be constructed.) I am not in a position to give a knockdown argument showing that the true and sufficiently complete christology is contradictory; having such arguments for any matter whatsoever is difficult, especially given our epistemic fallibility. What I offer here are seven (closely related) considerations that motivate a contradictory christology over its consistent competitors.[1]

Before turning to the seven virtues I should make one negative claim abundantly plain: I am *not* suggesting a contradictory approach as the last resort! Thomas McCall, in a very useful discussion of Contradictory Christology (McCall, 2019), suggests that we should turn to a contradictory account of Christ only if the quest for consistency is doomed. Why think that? McCall's discussion suggests that we should hold to the standard account – the mainstream account – of logical consequence unless we are clearly forced by a particular datum to reject it. But such thinking, in my view, is simply wrong. The mainstream account, as per §2, was drawn up as the correct account of logical consequence in mathematics. That's it. Now, one might argue that the right account of logical consequence in our true mathematical theories has to be the right account for all of our true theories

---

[1] I restrict attention, as throughout the book, to those christologies that not only contain Chalcedon 451 christology but also to those that involve a commitment to 'classical' accounts of divinity and humanity, even if, per some such accounts (e.g., §5.5.1), the given classical notions require revision to avoid contradiction.

The Contradictory Christ. Jc Beall, Oxford University Press (2021). © Jc Beall.
DOI: 10.1093/oso/9780198852360.003.0003

(despite the vastly richer languages involved in non-mathematical theories). I've seen no good argument along those lines. Pending such an argument, the position according to which the mainstream account of logic is the true account remains without good argument, at least for all that I can see.

What follows are seven directions of argument in favor of accepting a contradictory account of Christ.

3.1 Simplicity

Contradictory Christology, as I advance it, is the simplest account of the apparent contradiction of Christ: exactly 1 person who is 1 divine person (with all properties thereby entailed) who is also 1 human person (with all properties thereby entailed).[2] The simplest explanation of the apparent contradiction is that the appearance is veridical. Except when saddled with an incorrect account of logical consequence, the contradiction who is Christ is exactly what anyone would expect from taking the transcendence and boundlessness of the immutable and impeccable God and uniting – however mysteriously – with the immanent, bounded, mutable and peccable humanity with which we are so intimately familiar, uniting not in a way that results in two different persons or a new hybrid 'divine-human' nature, but uniting into exactly 1 person, who is 1 divine person who is also 1 human person.

One wishing to consistentize the apparent contradiction has many routes, from sophisticated accounts of 'persons', to sophisticated accounts of 'divine', to sophisticated accounts of 'human', to sophisticated accounts of the semantics of divine predicates or human predicates, to the many mereological and metaphysical maps of how the hypostatic union may be drawn, to so much more. But by my lights the simplest conclusion is the one drawn by multitudes of non-christian thinkers over the centuries, including the many

---

[2] Lest Nestorian red flags be thrown let me be plain: Christ is 1 human person in that Christ is a person and Christ is human. Rejecting that Christ is a human person is precisely one of the wrong directions against which Chalcedon firmly stands. After all, to be 1 human person is just to be 1 person who is human – *full stop*. Worries about Nestorian distortions can be good when the worries are well-founded but they can also distract from the simple but starkly powerful foundations of Chalcedonian creed: namely, that Christ is exactly 1 person who is divine (and so 1 divine person), exactly 1 person who is human (and so 1 human person), and exactly 1 person full stop – and therefore not two persons smashed together mysteriously or anything of the sort. (Note too that rejecting the claim that Christ is a human person can wobble into another imbalance against which Chalcedon firmly stands: namely, Apollinaris- or Eutyches-like views that seem to resist the 'full humanity' of the incarnate God.)

non-christian monotheistic relatives: namely, that the distinguishing mark of Christianity is its core contradictions in Christ. On this account, non-christian thinkers clearly see the contradiction of Christ; they simply reject it. The mark of Christians, on this simple account, is that via faith they accept the contradiction; they believe that Christ is God incarnate, 1 divine person who is also 1 human person and who remains exactly 1 person. Cluttering the core of christian theology with seemingly baroque constructions towards consistency helps nobody, certainly not the service of christian apologetics. (Few – probably *no* – objectors to the apparent contradiction of Christ seriously doubt that some consistent construction or other can be done with the right amount of metaphysical and/or semantical verve; but too often such constructions appear to be not only unduly baroque but ultimately changing the topic – an issue to which I return below.)

The first argument is just that: namely, that the simplest account of the apparent contradiction who is Christ is that the appearance is veridical. While simplicity is not by itself a full-proof – or fool-proof – guide to truth (Meyer, 1971), the argument from simplicity to Christ's contradictory being weighs very heavily in my own mind. But it is not the only consideration.

3.2 Avoiding ad hoc changes in meaning

In the quest to consistentize Christ a change-the-meaning strategy is common. One avenue along this route is to change the meaning of 'divine' and/or 'human', perhaps rejecting the so-called classic-theism account of divinity or, in the other direction, the classic conception of humanity. A directly related strategy is to change the meaning – the standard usage – of the fundamental-problem predicates such as 'mutable' and 'immutable' and so on. (Such explicit meaning changes are discussed under 'upstream' and 'downstream' meaning-change strategies in §5.)

By my lights, an unyielding quest for consistency makes these change-the-meanings strategies important avenues to pursue – and perhaps some may even be required by a particular conception of Catholicism (Pawl, 2016). Still, there is no question whatsoever that, independent of the quest to consistentize Christ, the change-the-meaning approach is ad hoc.

One might, of course, say that my account, which relies on a subclassical – and thereby non-classical, and thereby non-standard or otherwise non-mainstream – account of logic, is equally ad hoc. But that's wrong. My approach not only doesn't change the meaning of target divine and human predicates; it also doesn't change the meaning of the logical vocabulary. As §2 makes plain, exactly the standard truth and falsity conditions are given for logic's truth and falsity operators. Moreover, on my account exactly the standard satisfaction conditions for target divine and human predicates are intact.

3.3 Metaphysical neutrality

It strikes me as a very strong methodological principle that, in the absence of an officially revealed metaphysics, a metaphysically neutral solution to the fundamental 'problem' of christology – to the apparent contradiction of Christ – is better than one whose viability depends on the would-be truth of a specific metaphysical theory. Of course, every account of divinity, humanity, and whathaveyou involves some metaphysics or other; the point is that one's solution to the fundamental problem is better off than otherwise if it doesn't demand a particular metaphysics; rather, it is better off being neutral with respect to whatever the ultimate true metaphysics of such matters happens to be. (Again, this is in the absence of an officially revealed metaphysical theory.)

Contradictory Christology, as I've advanced it, is metaphysically neutral to a degree that consistent christologies do not approach. While philosophers and theologians hope to one day obtain the true metaphysics of 'persons', of 'wills', of 'natures' and so on (and so on), the viability of Contradictory Christology, as I've advanced it, is not threatened by the outcome of metaphysical inquiry. Such is very much not the case with many consistentizations of Christ; and I count this as a mark in favor of Contradictory Christology and against the consistentizations that turn on the fate of a particular metaphysical theory.

An example of what I take to be a loaded metaphysical solution – which, incidentally, is also a loaded 'semantic' solution – is the recent work of Pawl (2016). In particular, Pawl's proposed christology requires a so-called concretist account of the two natures of Christ; it requires that those subjects – the human nature of Christ and the divine nature of Christ – be the principal bearers of Christ's (ultimately derivative) divine and human properties.[3] Such a metaphysics is coherent; and such a metaphysical theory,

---

[3] In §5, I discuss the sense in which, on various QUA views and related compositional-like views, Christ's properties are 'derivative'.

together with Pawl's non-standard semantical theory, provides yet another consistent account of Christ's apparent contradiction. But at least from my perspective such a metaphysics looks to get its main motivation simply from the quest for consistency. By my lights, the given metaphysics may well be true (and, so, true regardless of christology); however, pending a clearly revealed account of the true metaphysics, a solution to the fundamental problem of christology – to the apparent contradiction at the core of christian theology – strikes me as worse off than otherwise if its viability turns on the truth of one particular metaphysical theory.

Pawl's particular metaphysics is just one of many (many) examples of would-be 'consistentizations' of christology that turn on a particular metaphysical theory. If either Christ or even the conciliar fathers (at least up through Chalcedon 451) had explicitly stamped a precise theory of metaphysics as the truth about metaphysics, and hadn't left the claims of Chalcedon to be in so many striking ways metaphysically neutral and apparently contradictory, I would not point to its metaphysical neutrality as an argument for Contradictory Christology. But, unless I missed something, there is no officially stamped christian metaphysics. The metaphysics of the true christian theology is the true metaphysics – full stop – just as the physics (biology, chemistry, mathematics, etc.) of true christian theology is simply the true physics (biology, chemistry, mathematics, etc.). As above, it strikes me as a strong methodological principle that, in the absence of an officially stamped revealed metaphysics, a metaphysically neutral account of the 'problem' of Christ's apparent contradictions is better than a metaphysically invested one.

3.4 Preserving the principal subject of christology

By my lights, the proposed contradictory account of Christ is not only simpler and metaphysically neutral compared with consistent accounts; it also keeps the principal subject of christology where it should be: namely, on Christ.

By all lights, except perhaps for those lights tinted by substantive theoretical commitments to particular solutions, a christology wherein Christ is the principal subject of Christ's properties is better than one wherein something that is not Christ is the principal subject of the key properties 'of Christ'. Despite this shared desideratum, the history of christology is peppered with proposals that shift the principal subject away from Christ. This issue is discussed further in §5, but a very short illustration of the issue concerns so-called reduplicative or, more simply, the QUA family of solutions.[4]

QUA solutions – if they don't engage in changing the meanings of expressions appearing in (for example) the fundamental-problem claims – ultimately reject the standard christological claims that generate the contradiction, replacing those claims with what are supposed to be close (but plainly non-contradictory) cousins involving some QUA device (e.g., 'According to divine nature', or 'insofar as divine', or 'as a divine being' or etc.). The salient avenues of such QUA accounts diverge on where the QUA device goes (and on what the QUA device ultimately means), but a natural and common one often looks as follows:[5]

1. Christ-qua-divine is impeccable.
2. Christ-qua-human is peccable.

One immediately asks: what is this entity called 'Christ-qua-human' (ditto 'Christ-qua-divine')? Who are these beings – the ones named, respectively, by 'Christ-qua-divine' and 'Christ-qua-human'? And most pressing of all: why are we talking about these entities when the issue on the table is that Christ – the one and only GodMan – is both impeccable and peccable (or mutable and immutable, or passible and impassible, etc.)?

Lest one think that the given questions have the same easy and obvious answer – namely, Christ the one and only GodMan – one point should be made plain: namely, that whatever (or even whomever) Christ-qua-human or Christ-qua-divine are, neither one is Christ. Suppose otherwise. Then we have the identity of Christ and Christ-qua-divine and, assuming that the target christological identity relation is transitive, we therefore also have the identity of Christ-qua-divine and Christ-qua-human.[6] But now the contradiction of Christ remains in plain view:

---

[4] I use 'QUA', spelled just so, to mention not only the various so-called reduplicative approaches that often use the word 'qua'; I also use it to mention the variety of linguistic devices that might be (and sometimes are) used instead of the word 'qua' (e.g., 'according to the divine [human] nature', 'in virtue of', 'as such', 'insofar as Christ is [divine/human]', and so on).

[5] QUA solutions often don't spell the singular term – the Subject term, the principal name – with hyphens; however, spelling it just so is perfectly in line with the QUA position, and is perhaps less misleading than dropping the hyphen, as Senor (2002) makes plain.

[6] §5 discusses the would-be promise of so-called relative-identity accounts of identity relations, ones that may (though don't always) undermine the given transitivity of the relation. §6 discusses a non-transitive theology identity relation involved in the trinity.

1. Christ (who just is Christ-qua-divine) is impeccable.
2. Christ (who just is Christ-qua-human) is peccable.
3. Christ is both peccable and impeccable.

Since the QUA solutions are one and all on the quest to consistentize Christ, and the target QUA solutions reject change-the-meanings strategies (e.g., changing the meanings of 'impeccable' or 'peccable' so as to avoid their jointly entailed contradiction), said QUA solutions reject that Christ is either Christ-qua-divine or Christ-qua-human.

And so the questions remain: What are these beings? Who are these beings? And why are we talking about *their* being impeccable and/or peccable when the principal subject of our concern is Christ's peccability and impeccability?

A natural reply is that Christ-qua-human and Christ-qua-divine are the fundamental and principal bearers of the given properties: these are the subjects of mutability and immutability (and so on), not Christ himself. Christ gets to count as having such properties only by charity; he – Christ – does not in fact exemplify any of the target properties.

More on this topic needs to be said, and a bit more is said in §4 and §5. For present considerations, the key point is that some attempts to consistentize Christ ultimately reject that Christ is the bearer of the target properties, shifting the focus instead to the principal subjects of such properties – different subjects that ultimately bear the awesome weight of the contrary properties that Christ would otherwise have to bear only by being a contradictory being. Such a shift, as discussed again in §5, strikes me as a step in the wrong direction, at least if one takes seriously the very live option of Christ's being a contradictory being.

3.5 Balancing 'from above' and 'from below'

Theologians face a longstanding struggle to balance the humanity and divinity of Christ. One (of many many many) illustrations of this involves debates about Christ's divine-vs-human properties. Oliver Crisp's discussion of 'impeccable versus merely sinless' nicely reflects the situation (Crisp, 2009), a struggle to respect all divine properties of Christ (including impeccability) and all human properties of Christ (including, many think, peccability). As Crisp's discussion makes clear, a christology imbalanced 'from above' falls prey to a distortion of Christ's genuine humanity, including

Christ's genuine human experiences – the experiences as we, in our limited and peccable state, experience them. On this threat Crisp quotes Trevor Hart:

> If we draw that line in such a way that it removes from Jesus all possibility of sinning, are we not thereby precisely robbing him of the experience of 'being tempted in all things as we are'? Is the genuine potential for sin not analytic in some way in the very notion of temptation? Certainly it would seem to be basic to human temptation as we know and experience it.
>
> (Hart, 1995, p. 38)

One is drawn, then, towards rebalancing the christology 'from below', to fully embrace the peccability of Christ. But hold on! Christ is God; and God is wholly good – and therefore wholly impeccable. As Crisp makes plain, in response to the potentially dangerous shifting of weights, one must avoid an imbalance 'from below':

> If God is necessarily good – a view that is certainly deeply ingrained in Christian theology and spirituality, to the extent that it is the default view in the tradition – then . . . he cannot be able to sin. . . . [O]ne could simply stipulate that God is not necessarily good in some sense, but this is surely indicative of the theological dilettante.   (Crisp, 2009, p. 135)

Hence, argues Crisp, Christ is impeccable. But, now, hold on! Christ is human – as human as you and me. Therefore, even apart from the demands of 'experiencing as we experience' (see Hart quote above), Christ's humanity involves peccability. Christ is sinless, without question; however, Christ is human and so peccable. To reject Christ's peccability is to diminish Christ's humanity – or so the apparent pull 'from below' tugs.

What to do? What the true (Chalcedon-constrained) christology demands seems to be perfect balance. Indeed, perfect balance is precisely the reason for the qualifiers 'fully divine' and 'fully human' (as opposed to an imbalanced 'mostly divine' or 'mostly human', etc.). On the longstanding issue of whether Christ is peccable or 'merely sinless', achieving perfect balance seems to demand a contradiction: namely, that Christ is impeccable (because Christ is God) and Christ is peccable (because Christ is human). But unless one shifts standard meanings of the terms, or perhaps shifts the principal subject of the given properties, or perhaps both, the apparent contradiction is genuine: namely, that it's both true and false that Christ is impeccable.

Crisp's solution is to reject the contradiction – and the perfect balance – in favor of 'above'. Crisp's account tries to accommodate the concerns 'from below', but ultimately it's plain (I think) that the resulting imbalance is unsatisfactory, at least when the contradictory option is plainly available. To accommodate the concerns 'from below' Crisp suggests that Christ 'qua human' is peccable but the peccability, in effect, is neutralized by Christ 'qua divine'. In short, we have a case where Christ *could* sin if it weren't for the impenetrable protective barricade provided by *Christ qua divine*. Such a solution to the apparent contradiction is intriguing and certainly consistent (as far as it goes); but it fails to accommodate the demands 'from below' that it purports to address. After all, on this account, Christ knows that *Christ qua human* can never succumb to sin. How is this remotely the same experience as our experience in the face of temptation and sin more generally? It isn't. Ultimately, Crisp's solution tilts in favor 'of above' in an effort to avoid the otherwise contradictory Christ. Christ isn't really peccable; it's just, once again, Christ-qua-human to which 'peccability' applies.

Of course, the issue of (im-) peccability is one of many, many examples of the apparent contradiction brought about by Christ's 'fully balanced' human-ity and divinity. And beyond Crisp's discussion there are many (many) other examples of trying – but, from what I can see, failing – to achieve the balance of Christ's 'full humanity' and 'full divinity'. That there are many failures is not surprising: the only way to completely balance the two is contradictory. The quest to consistentize the apparent contradiction of Christ is inevitably doomed to an imbalanced account.

3.6 Preserving the mystery of the hypostatic union

The quest for a consistent characterization of Christ is one that faces a challenge: namely, the mystery of the hypostatic union. On the surface, it's the apparent contradiction of Christ which fuels the mystery. Nobody, so far as I can tell, thinks that there's some special problem in God's uniting two natures (perhaps more natures) into one person. The problem, rather, concerns the specific (contradiction-entailing) natures in question. Uniting the divine nature and the human nature into one fully divine and fully human person looks to be a contradictory crossing: a crossing poeticized over centuries as the one transcendent God against the one *and same* God on the cross; a crossing stamped in the creeds of God's hanging in atonement while being free from all constraint; a contradictory crossing that screams out for a consistent way to characterize the apparent crossing – perhaps two distinct persons are involved? or two distinct gods? or only an apparent human apparently hanging on the cross? or so on or so on or so on through every combinatorial consistentization imaginable. But if, per the longstanding quest, the hypostatic union is in fact consistent then wherein lies the mystery? On every consistent account of Christ's apparent contradiction I, for one (but I doubt I'm alone), find myself at a loss to understand wherein the mystery is supposed to lie – except for the general mystery that permeates all of God's actions, but not anything peculiar to the hypostatic union. Of course, on each such consistentization of Christ's apparent contradictions the account comes with official fine print: namely, a claim that the full truth remains mysterious. But, again, except for God's mystery in general, wherein the specific mystery is supposed to lie in such consistentizations of Christ remains very much unclear.

A contradictory christology manifests the mystery in ways that are unavailable (or, at least, unnatural) to any of the consistentized accounts. On my contradictory christology the mystery is not *that* Christ is contradictory; for *that*, after all, is just the clear and obvious starting line – the clear and pressing 'problem' with which we all begin. The mystery is rather one of implementation or mechanism: *how* the contradiction was pulled off. We have precise (largely mathematical) models of how to think about the contradiction; but these models are at best guides to the truths that follow (or don't follow) from Christ's contradictory being; they don't provide an explanation of how the actual contradiction was realized. How a contradiction is truly realized in a world that in most other respects is truly described by consistent theories remains mysterious at its core.

3.7 Christology and the obvious need for faith

A solution to the fundamental problem should naturally reflect why faith in Christ – faith in the incarnate God – is necessary. A contradictory christology promises a natural and intriguing explanation of the necessity of faith. Along these lines, one explanation might be that at least some (if not all) of the contradictory truths of Christ – God's incarnate revelation and gift of atonement – are literally incredible.

In what sense might the contradictions of Christ be literally incredible? Let us say that a logical conjunction $A \wedge B$ is *fully believable at time t* just if the conjunction and both conjuncts are believable at time t. (Of course, this is restricted to a fixed believer/agent.) It may be – though I need to emphasize that I am not hereby committing to the claim – that few gluts (few true contradictions) are fully believable in the given sense. In particular, it may be that there is no contradiction which is both true of Christ and fully believable by any non-divine being. The truth of Christ, I say, is contradictory. Believing the full truth requires believing the contradictions true of Christ. In practice, Christians often feel the sheer difficulty of believing the contradiction of Christ's 'full divinity and full humanity', at least at a particular time. The difficulty is not for want of commitment or some lamentable 'backsliding' or the like. It's a deeper difficulty the very root of which lies in the incarnation. In practice, Christians often find times when they rely on the truth of Christ's divine properties while resting on the falsity of Christ's human properties; and at other times Christians rely on the falsity of Christ's divine properties while resting on the truth of Christ's human properties. The push-and-pull between Christ's human properties and Christ's divine properties is precisely the fuel behind many historical heresies and subsequently many crises of faith. In mystic traditions (not that I'm an expert), reaching a state of spiritual insight requires the seemingly impossible *full belief*; it requires simultaneously believing contradictory claims of Christ.

I am not in any way suggesting that the right direction for christology is mysticism. I am *not* suggesting that. (I wouldn't even know what that amounts to, frankly.) What I am suggesting is that a systematic christology that makes obvious the need for faith is better off than one that doesn't. And while each and every consistentized christology can find ways to accommodate the in-practice data (e.g., Christians don't rest on the falsity of Christ's divine properties but rather they at times just ignore them, or whathaveyou), I think that a contradictory christology might be best positioned to naturally reflect the requirement of faith. By my lights, the requirement of faith is best rooted in the incarnation itself: faith that Christ is the transcendent God and that Christ is as human as you and me, peccable as we are, impeccable as God must be – and not because of some secretively non-standard semantics or the like. On my view, the contradictions involved in the incarnation, so understood, may not be 'fully believable' in the sense above, and precisely in that respect *faith* in the contradictions of Christ – faith in the contradiction who is Christ – is obviously required.

But let me be clear: much more needs to be thought about here. Reason Seven for a contradictory christology remains budding in ways that the other six considerations do not. But buds, at least in this case, are not without promise and not without force.

** *Parenthetical note.* I must emphasize that Contradictory Christology, as I'm advancing it, is *not* committed to explaining the necessity of faith in these terms. The foregoing remarks offer an intriguing and in some ways natural explanation open to a contradictory christology; they are not necessitated by any contradictory christology. Moreover, I should also emphasize that nothing I've said here is intended to address debates about the would-be equivalence between *faith* and *saving faith*. (Thanks to Jonathan Rutledge for flagging this clarification.) *End note.* **

3.8 Closing big-picture remarks

It seems to me plain as day that christian theologians who aim to embrace the striking Chalcedon 'axioms' of Christ have been pursuing consistency at the cost of the simple but striking truth: namely, that the incarnation really is as contradictory as it appears. Clinging to consistency has produced a multitude of metaphysical gadgets and baroque edifices; but each such construction, while interesting and abstractly coherent, always carries the whiff of heresy – more divine than human, more human than divine, seemingly two persons even if the officially proffered account squints to find but one, and/or so on and so on. At every turn the quest for a consistent account of Christ appears to focus too much 'from below' or too much 'from above'. And so on.

What distinguishes the christian account from its traditional monotheistic cousins is precisely the apparent contradiction at its core:[7] the union of the divine and human, the union of the transcendent and immanent, the union of the infinite god and the finite human, the union of the sacred and the mundane. Such a union is not even remotely contradictory or even mildly paradoxical if the result of the union involves two persons, or involves a god in human form but not a genuine human, or involves a human but not genuinely a god, or so on. No, the striking and radical core of the christian account of reality is the palpable contradiction imprinted at Chalcedon: exactly one person, who is as divine as any divine person and who is as human as any human person.

The standard reaction to such an apparently contradictory characterization of the core of christian theology is clear and constant: the characterization is either nonsense (because inconsistent) or its consistency rests on some elaborate metaphysical or semantical construction. And so we go: rejecting

---

[7] The trinity, of course, is also distinctive, a topic I touch on in the final chapter (viz., §6).

the inconsistency on apparent pain of nonsense or going to the metaphysical or semantical toolshed to construct some wedge through which some sort of consistent account may fit.

I say that the apparent struggle is not only unnecessary; it's a dangerous one that takes its adherents further and further away from the simple – though gobsmacking – core truth: the contradictory Christ.

As I said in §1, non-christian thinkers have in many ways seen the crux of christian theology very clearly, perhaps even more clearly than Christians; they've seen that the story that Christians are telling – the union of 'above' and 'below' into exactly one person with the nature of 'above' and also the full nature of 'below' (our nature) – entails a contradiction. And it's precisely that contradiction – whom Christians recognize as Messiah, Redeemer, and Lord – that repels so many, including, alas, the very thinkers and christian theologians who should openly embrace the contradiction. Building elaborate 'secret' or hidden constructs that might consistentize the contradiction away – the contradiction who is Christ – has long been understandable given standard thinking about logic. But it has also, for just that long, been a march in the wrong direction.

The core of christian theology is a contradiction; the right response is to make sense of it, not flee from it. Shake the dogma that all inconsistent theories should be rejected, and then pause to reflect: might Christ, in his persistent appearance of contradictory properties, be contradictory – truly contradictory? I say: yes.

4

Some objections

With the central core of Contradictory Christology in place, together with at least seven considerations towards Contradictory Christology, this chapter elaborates the account by replying to a wide range of objections and questions.

The objections and replies are loosely and only very crudely categorized into five groups, none sitting perfectly well under its given tag but sitting well enough for purposes of covering the issues. The five groups are: methodological issues, epistemological issues, theological issues, metaphysical issues (with a very generous remit for metaphysics), and, for lack of a better term, ecumenical issues. The chapter simply marches through target objections and questions, giving my responses to each in turn.[1]

4.1 Methodological issues

4.1.1 Your theology is false!

Your christology (and theology, more generally) has it that various central christian claims are both true and false, and therefore false! Your account of Christ is therefore false. Therefore, we should reject your account.[2]

Reply. Any sentence or theory which is both true and false is false – and, notably, true. To reject a truth because it is also false is to reject a truth – and thereby reject part of the full truth of the given part of reality. By my lights, the project of giving the full truth of reality – in this case, the full theological truth – is the goal. For most parts of reality, there's no persistent appearance of inconsistency or contradiction, and so the project of giving the full truth

---

[1] Much (though not all) of this chapter overlaps with or otherwise is taken directly from material in my symposium papers in the *Journal of Analytic Theology* (Beall *et al.*, 2019).

[2] Compare Tuggy (2011, para. 2, fn. 2).

The Contradictory Christ. Jc Beall, Oxford University Press (2021). © Jc Beall.
DOI: 10.1093/oso/9780198852360.003.0004

typically goes hand in hand with giving only the truth (so to speak) – the project of having no false sentences in our account. But that's most parts of reality; Christ is clearly very different, a case in which, as Tuggy (2011, p. 206) puts it, '[a]ble and responsible thinkers squarely face the appearance of contradiction [in Christ].' Given that reality itself is contradictory – that there is a contradictory being in reality – the true account of reality is itself contradictory, and thereby false in addition to being true. Why, then, should we reject the true account, as the given objection charges? Pending a good answer, I suggest that we reject the call for rejection, and accept the full truth, contradictory as it is. A false theory should be rejected unless doing so precludes accepting the full truth.

4.1.2 Truth requires coherence

Coherence is a necessary condition for truth, and a coherent christology rules out Contradictory Christology since a *true list of Christ's properties cannot contain contradictory pairs*.[3]

Reply. Setting aside epistemic and question-begging accounts of 'coherence' (as, respectively, irrelevant and uncharitable) the objection rests on a true principle: namely, that true theories must 'hang together' in a way that avoids outright triviality, where triviality is the uncontroversially absurd 'trivial theory' – namely, the theory containing *all* sentences in the language of the theory.[4] On the standard view of logic no logically contradictory theory can 'hang together' (cohere) in the given way, since logic itself – on the standard view – takes every logically contradictory theory to the trivial theory. But that view of logic is not forced on theology; a more natural account of logic is available, as in §2. While true theories demand coherence, a logically contradictory theory can be coherent, contrary to the objection's presupposition.

---

[3] While he is not focused on a contradictory christology in the relevant passage, I frame the current objection in terms drawn from Richard Cross' state-of-debate discussion of the fundamental problem (Cross, 2011, p. 480).

[4] For example, the standard (say) theory of arithmetic (say, Peano Arithmetic) is written in a certain language, namely, the language of the theory; and the trivial theory of arithmetic, relative to that language, is the theory that contains all sentences of the language. (There is absolutely nothing special about arithmetic. It's used here as a very simple example of the term 'trivial theory' as it occurs in contemporary philosophy of logic.)

4.1.3 Uckelman's dilemma

Uckelman (2019) raises a dilemma for the very roots of Contradictory Christology. The dilemma:

> [E]ither Christology is not genuinely contradictory on the account of logical consequence that Beall advocates [viz., FDE] *or* if it is then switching to FDE doesn't help solve anything.   (Uckelman, 2019)

If Uckelman's dilemma is a genuine dilemma then Contradictory Christology must be rejected.

Reply. The dilemma is merely apparent.[5] Before explicitly taking each horn in turn, Uckelman's key notion of *genuinely contradictory* should be defined. As I understand her position, a sentence A, in the language of theory T, is *genuinely contradictory* iff A is explosive according to T, that is, iff according to theory T's entailment (consequence) relation, A entails all sentences in the language of T. In general, a genuinely contradictory sentence, on Uckelman's target usage, is either a theory-specific explosive sentence (i.e., a sentence in some true theory T which explodes according to T's consequence relation) or is a 'super-explosive sentence' – explodes on all consequence relations of any true theory. Generalizing to theories, a *theory* is *genuinely contradictory*, on Uckelman's target usage, just if it contains a genuinely contradictory sentence – and, hence, only if it's the given trivial theory.

Uckelman's first horn.
Uckelman's first horn is that the true christology is not genuinely contradictory according to its consequence relation. The problem, if I understand it correctly, is supposed to be that Contradictory Christology is *rightly* so called only if the advanced Christology is genuinely contradictory – in Uckelman's sense.

My reply to the first horn: I reject that Uckelman's sense of 'genuinely contradictory' is the only sense of the term that warrants the tag 'Contradictory

---

[5] I note, only tangentially, that in the background Uckelman assumes that either the true christology is contradictory – or *genuinely contradictory* (more on which below) – or it's false that the true christology is contradictory. I grant this particular (excluded-middle-ish) assumption, though I note that, on my view, logic itself doesn't demand it.

Christology'. After all, there is a clear and well-established sense in which a theory is genuinely contradictory if it contains a contradiction, and containing a sentence of the form *it is true that p and it's false that p* is certainly a well-established way to contain a contradiction. True, such contradictions do not explode according to logic (i.e., according to what I take to be the true account of logical consequence); but they remain true and false, and that's a well-worn way of being contradictory – since being true and false is sufficient for the truth of the corresponding contradiction. (Stretching out the point: if you're true, then so too is an application of logic's truth operator to you; but if you're false, then an application of the dual of logic's truth operator – namely, its falsity operator (viz., logical negation) – is true; and, finally, the logical conjunction of those two truths is thereby true too. But since the given true conjunction has false conjuncts, the conjunction itself is false too. And all of that appears to be contradictory – and genuinely so – on very well-worn uses of the term.)

On my account of logic (-al consequence) *no* sentence is 'genuinely contradictory' in Uckelman's sense, given that there's no sentence that is explosive according to logic itself. By my lights, this is in fact a virtue of the account of logic (-al consequence); it reflects a purity of topic-neutrality in the sense that, on the given account, logic takes no stand on the truth of elementary truth/falsity attributions – no stand on the status of $\dagger p$ or $\neg p$ for arbitrary (logically atomic) p in any possibility recognized by logic (i.e., any logical possibility, the ones over which logical consequence is defined). But putting the account of logic (and its virtues) aside, Uckelman's first horn fails to have its intended point: it is not a bad result that the true christology isn't 'genuinely contradictory' in Uckelman's sense; but since my proposed Contradictory Christology remains contradictory in other clear senses the tag 'Contradictory Christology' remains warranted.

** *Parenthetical remark.* Perhaps worth flagging is that in the end I don't terribly much care about the terminology, and so if Uckelman's super contradictions (as I call them above) – or individually theory-specific explosive sentences – are the only 'genuine contradictions', fine; I'm not then advancing a genuinely contradictory theology because I'm not advancing the trivial theology. But as far as I can see, the wider debates around glut theory and would-be true negation-inconsistent theories favor (or at least clearly ground) the usage I've employed in this book and elsewhere (Beall, 2009). *End remark.* **

Uckelman's second horn.
Uckelman's second horn is that my account of logic does nothing to save a genuinely contradictory theory – *in Uckelman's sense* – from absurdity.

My reply to the second horn: Uckelman is right. If the true theology – or any true theory – were to be 'genuinely contradictory' in Uckelman's sense then some trivial theory would be true, and we all recognize that 'possibility' as both the mark of absurdity and a mark against which we all rationally run. But, again, the sharpness of this horn in the would-be dilemma is little (to nil); there is no suggestion that Contradictory Christology contains explosive sentences. And, again, that it must contain them on pain of being badly named (or worse) is a claim the force of which I do not see.

4.1.4 The 'loss' of material modus ponens and more

The given Contradictory Christology takes logical consequence to be per the FDE account as advanced in §2. Hence, on the given account, we lose the logical validity of material modus ponens, material modus tollens, and disjunctive syllogism, where these can be thought of as 'argument forms' or sentence-sentence or set-sentence forms (where the set contains only sentences). Let $\rightarrow$ be logic's material conditional, defined (per usual) via logical negation and logical disjunction:

$$A \rightarrow B := \neg A \vee B$$

The given argument forms are

- Material Modus Ponens (MMP): $A, A \rightarrow B \therefore B$
- Material Modus Tollens (MMT): $\neg A, B \rightarrow A \therefore \neg B$
- Disjunctive Syllogism (DS): $\neg A, A \vee B \therefore B$

Each of these forms is logically invalid on the going account of logical consequence. A single counterexample, which exists in logic's space of possibilities, refutes their would-be logical validity: namely, a case in which A is a glut and B is gap (i.e., not at least true and not at least false).[6] Since

---

[6] Counterexamples for each of the given forms can be given without invoking gaps but using gaps affords a single counterexample to all three.

A is (at least) true (since glutty), so too is the logical disjunction of *A* and any sentence in the language, including *B* and including the negation of *B*, namely ¬*B*. But, then, each of *A* ∨ *B* and ¬*B* ∨ *A* are (at least) true, in which case, by definition of the material conditional, *B* → *A* is (at least true). But since *B* is a gap, neither *B* nor its negation ¬*B* is true in the given case, and hence none of the conclusions in the target forms are even at least true. This refutes the would-be logical validity of MMT and DS. To see that MMP is similarly refuted, note that since *A* is a glut, its negation ¬*A* is also true; and, hence, by truth conditions for disjunctions ¬*A* ∨ *B* is at least true, and hence by definition of the material conditional *A* → *B* is at least true; ergo, the second premise of MPP is at least true; ergo, from this and above, both premises of MPP are at least true, but *B*, being a gap, is not even at least true.

The objection is that rejecting the logical validity of such common patterns is too much to lose; their apparent ubiquity in true theories is undeniable. Accommodating the alleged contradictions of Christ by losing so very much of logical entailment is to lose too much for responsible theorizing.

Reply. The claim that my account of logical consequence rejects the logical validity of such common forms is exactly right. But is this a loss? Well, logic never validated them; rather, a bad account of logic validated them. The pressing question is what to make of the apparent ubiquity of such argument forms that appear to underwrite our 'reasoning' and the consequence relations involved in many, many, many of our true theories? Without an answer to this, Contradictory Christology appears to be plainly implausible: we're left with next to no resources to do our theology (or, for that matter, biology, physics, mathematics, more)!

This issue is a very big one. (And that's an understatement.) This book is not the venue to tackle the problem, but let me highlight some important directions of reply that, by my lights, sufficiently address the concerns.

4.1.4.1 Extra-logical consequence and logical vocabulary
One important reply is that in many of our true theories we are not dealing with glutty (i.e., contradictory) phenomena; the theories rule out the logical possibility of gluts as theoretical impossibilities. But take away the theoretical possibility of gluts, so that a theory's entailment (consequence) relation doesn't treat them as candidate counterexamples, and you've thereby taken away the common core of the (logical) counterexamples to MPP, MTT, and DS. Accordingly, those forms are valid according to the given theories that restrict the space of available possibilities. And this is precisely what happens

in our true theory of (for example) arithmetic, biology or so on. In particular, even though

$$A, A \rightarrow B \therefore B$$

is *logically* invalid, it is valid according to those consequence relations involved in true theories whose space of possibilities precludes (the logical possibilitiy of) gluts.

The details of how this is pulled off are less pressing than that it is pulled off in many true theories.[7] In turn, the explanation for why so many of our true theories appear to validate MMP, MMT, and DS – where these use only logic's given expressions (i.e., logic's conditional, negation, etc.) – is that they do validate MMP, MMT, and DS. Logic itself doesn't do the work for the theories; the theories' respective consequence relations build in extra-logical (and otherwise logically invalid) patterns that result in the given theory-specific validities.

4.1.4.2 Extra-logical vocabulary

Another important reply is that while the logical invalidity of MMP, MMT, and DS may be initially surprising, the effects of such logical invalidity are minor-to-nil, even if extra-logical consequence relations (per §4.1.4.1) are set aside. On this reply, one points not (mainly) to extra-logical constraints imposed on a theory's consequence relations; instead, one points to extra-logical vocabulary for which modus ponens, modus tollens, even disjunctive syllogism are valid (according to any entailment relation defined over that vocabulary). Skipping details here, the idea is simply that there are more conditionals involved in many of our true theories than logic's material conditional; and it may well be that modus ponens for such conditionals is not in any way undermined by the possibility of gluts. Similarly, mutatis mutandis, for different negations and disjunctions.

On this direction of reply, the widespread appearance of MMP's validity, MTT's validity and so on is one of mistaken identity: the expressions involved aren't in fact logic's expressions (for which such forms are invalid) but rather extra-logical vocabulary for which such forms are valid.[8]

---

[7] For some details see, for example, my papers on 'shrieking' and, similarly, 'shrugging' (Beall, 2013*b,c*, 2018).

[8] For details on this sort of reply, see the work of early 'relevance' (aka 'relevant') logicians Anderson *et al.* (1992); Routley *et al.* (1982) and various applications (Beall, 2009; Field, 2008; Priest, 2006). References in such works point to a multitude of other works in which such ideas are discussed.

4.1.4.3 Necessary instances versus valid forms

Yet another reply is that MMP and so on have counterexamples even though many of its instances don't. In particular, it might be, as a matter of fact, that the vast majority of *instances* of MMP are necessarily truth-preserving over all relevant possibilities even though, of course, there are a few instances that spoil the soup (so to say). On this reply, we are surprised to learn that MMP (etc.) is logically invalid because the vast majority of instances of MMP are necessarily true across the space of all possibilities that wind up being theoretically possible (according to our true theories).[9]

4.1.4.4 Theory-specific absurdities and 'DS' etc.

Another sort of reply, similar to some of the foregoing, is another case of mistaken identity. In this case, we are in fact relying on theory-specific absurdities when we 'reason' in disjunctive-syllogism or 'reductio' sorts of ways. Consider one example, where $\vdash_T$ is the consequence relation of theory T, and $\perp$ is some T-specific absurdity, some explosive sentence according to $\vdash_T$ where, let us stipulate (for simplicity), $\perp$ is (just) false in every possibility (model) recognized by $\vdash_T$. In this case, we have the sort of reductio- or disjunctive-syllogism-like pattern:

- If $A \vdash_T \perp$ (i.e., A entails an absurdity) and $A \lor B$ is true according to T, then either B is true according to T or T is the trivial theory (for the given language).

The idea here is that this sort of reductio- or disjunctive-syllogism-like pattern is ultimately the only sort of such pattern that we ever need in our theorizing. The given pattern (or, if you want, principle) might not – for various technical reasons – be expressible in the target theory T to which the principle applies; but it's a prevalent principle for reasoning about T.

4.1.4.5 Extra-linguistic acceptance–rejection

One other reply (probably not the last available) points not to extra-logical consequence relations, which beef up entailment relations to validate MMP etc., and points not to extra-logical vocabulary to stand in for the otherwise weak (but universal) logical vocabulary, but rather points to 'extra-linguistic' behavior that we – qua theorists – utilize in our reasoning about theories. The details of this reply are spelled out in different ways in different places, but

---

[9] This sort of story is gestured at in my *Spandrels of Truth* book (Beall, 2009).

the basic idea is that when we talk about the apparent validity of MMP (or the like) we are instead talking about rational acceptance–rejection behavior, whereby we have both of the following sentences

$$A, A \rightarrow B$$

in our theory. Logic, of course, does not validate B's going into the theory; however, a generalization of logic (to so-called multiple-conclusion logic) does say that, where $!A$ is $A \wedge \neg A$ (as throughout the book), at least one of

$$!A, B$$

is true if our theory, which contains both A and $A \rightarrow B$, is itself true. Hence, if – for whatever our theoretical reasons – we reject the logical possibility of $!A$ (i.e., the possibility of the contradiction $A \wedge \neg A$ being true) we are then assured, by the given generalization of logic, that our putting B into the theory results in a theory which remains true.[10]

4.1.5 Gaps and gluts and Contradictory Christology

Cotnoir (2019) raises a challenge specifically towards the question of which candidate relation plays the role of logic – plays the role of universal consequence (closure) in all true theories. The answer I give, as discussed in §2, is FDE. But Cotnoir (2019, §3.2) argues that my account of logic is right only if my account of the true christology (and true theology more generally) is wrong. The argument points to the following claims:

C1. It is both true and false that Christ is immutable.
C2. It is neither true nor false that Christ is immutable.

My account of christology is committed to C1. Cotnoir points out that in light of containing C1 the true christology, one would expect, should not contain C2. But – and here's Cotnoir's given challenge – an FDE-sourced account of the vocabulary in C1 and C2 results in their (logical) equivalence. That this is so is explained as follows.

---

[10] Details of this sort of reply are filled out in various places, including especially Beall 2015 but also with important early ideas in Priest 2006.

An FDE-sourced account of C1 and C2 treats the phrases 'both true and false' and 'neither true nor false' as involving logical vocabulary – namely, logic's truth connective (viz., $\dagger$), logic's falsity connective (viz., $\neg$), logic's conjunction connective (viz., $\wedge$) and logic's disjunction connective (viz., $\vee$). In particular, where we can let C be 'Christ is immutable', an FDE-sourced account of C1's so-called form is

$$\dagger C \wedge \neg C$$

while an FDE-sourced account of C2's form is

$$\neg(\dagger C \vee \neg C)$$

Since logic's truth operator is (logically) redundant, the given forms for C1 and C2 are equivalent to

$$C \wedge \neg C$$

and, respectively,

$$\neg(C \vee \neg C)$$

And now Cotnoir's challenge comes to its point: according to FDE the given forms are logically equivalent! Hence, argues Cotnoir, since C1 is in the given christology so too is C2; but, Cotnoir suggests, C2 should not be in any christology that contains C1; and hence we should reject the account of logic underwriting the given christology.

Reply. This is an important issue but my reply is fairly straightforward. To begin, if – as Cotnoir suggests – we expect to reject C2 in the face of accepting C1 then our expectation belies an FDE-sourced reading of C1 and C2. Logical vocabulary is not in the business of making robust or substantive semantic claims; its vocabulary is topic-neutral, and in many ways non-explanatory.[11] But as Cotnoir's expressed expectation reveals, the idea of a sentence being both true and false – if important or explanatory –

---

[11] My own view of logic's truth and falsity operators is that they are the source of so-called deflationary views of corresponding truth and falsity predicates, which are not explanatory in any interesting ways (Beall, 2019b).

is not equivalent to a sentence being neither true nor false. What, then, is the non-FDE-sourced form of C1 and C2? The answer involves an explanatory notion of gluts and gaps; and my own view is that such notions are to be expressed using theory-specific vocabulary; such notions do not – as the given expectations reveal – reduce to (non-explanatory) logical ingredients.

Details of the given theory-specific *glut* and *gap* predicates are important, but not for present purposes. For present purposes what's important is to see that Cotnoir's argument against an FDE-based contradictory christology fails: its premise that the forms of C1 and C2 are simply FDE-sourced clashes with the expectations imposed on C1 and C2.

4.1.6 Ad hoc

Contradictory Christology is ad hoc. The fundamental problem of christology is a difficult one to solve. The proposed contradictory account points to an alternative logic that can handle contradictions without reducing the theory to all-out absurdity, and then the proposal simply hitches the logic to christology without independent motivation.

Reply. This objection is misplaced on two fronts. To begin, my alternative account of logic has been motivated in the philosophy of logic by a very wide range of theology-independent phenomena, from concerns peculiar to 'relevance' of logic (Anderson and Belnap, 1975; Anderson et al., 1992) to modeling various inconsistent but not flat-out absurd theories (e.g., so-called naive account of sets or properties) to a host of strange phenomena from language (Priest, 2000). So, against the current objection, the given account of logic is not ad hoc.

The second front on which the objection is misplaced is the charge specific to christology, namely, that Contradictory Christology is an ad hoc solution to the fundamental problem. This is simply wrong. The very conciliar texts that at least in part define orthodox christology (and theology more generally) carry the prima facie contradiction of Christ on their jackets. That the true christology is in fact logically contradictory is a natural response to the fundamental problem; it has been long ignored simply because of a restricted account of logic.

4.2 Epistemological issues

4.2.1 From some to all contradictions

Once we accept some contradictions we have no grounds to reject any contradictions.

Reply. This is unmotivated. Consider the directly analogous claim: once we admit that quantum reality is funny we have no grounds to reject that all of reality is funny. Belaboring the reply (because the objection seems to be very common), consider another analogous claim (familiar to philosophers): once we accept that 'intersubstitutability of identicals' – or 'intersubstitutability of co-referential terms' – fails in some (true) theories we have no grounds to accept such intersubstitutability for any (true) theory. Again, this is simply unmotivated. When philosophers discovered so-called intensional or opaque contexts (e.g., *It is believed that...*), contexts in which all of the following are true for some names '*a*' and '*b*' and some predicate '*F*', they were surprised:[12]

- *a* is identical to *b*.
- It's true that So-n-so believes that *a* is *F*.
- It's false that (one and the same) So-n-so believes that *b* is *F*.

But the lesson is not that we now (i.e., post-discovery) have no reason to accept the intersubstitutability of identicals (or co-referential terms) in any true theory at all; the lesson is simply that there are true theories that accommodate peculiar contexts in which intersubstitutability fails. Finding unexpected, abnormal contexts in which intersubstitutability fails does not undermine the importance of such intersubstitutability in many (perhaps most) true theories. Of course, we were mistaken if we thought that the principle was logical and hence was thereby required across all true theories. Still, for all I can see, there is no reason not to demand such intersubstitutability in most of our true theories provided that the discovered (opaque)

---

[12] For a concrete example, replace '*a*' and '*b*' with 'Superman' and 'Clark Kent', respectively, and replace '*F*' with 'flying'. (And to make it doubly concrete, replace the general operator 'it is believed that...' with (for example) 'Lois Lane believes that....') For many more examples see the (vast) literature on intensional and/or opaque contexts.

contexts aren't in play (in the language of the theory). That we have found some contexts (or predicates) – or some phenomena – for which the given intersubstitutability fails gives no reason to reject the principle in (for example) our true theory of arithmetic, physics, or biology.

Contradictory Christology – and contradictory christian theology in general – is similar. We were mistaken in what we took to be a *logical* – and thereby absolutely universal – proscription against true contradictory theories. Still, for all that I can see, the candidates for true contradictory theories remain very rare – indeed, unique if we ignore 'spandrels of truth' (e.g., liar paradoxes, etc.). Of course, maybe the contradiction who is Christ is not unique; maybe there are other such contradictory beings; logic itself doesn't rule them out. But logic rules out precious little; and its failing to rule something out is hardly a good reason to accept it as a leading candidate for truth. (Otherwise, we have good reason to accept that pigs fly.) Until there's good reason to accept that our true theories of phenomena beyond Christ are likewise glutty I see no reason not to reject the spread of contradictory theories.

4.2.2 Which contradictions are true?

McCall (2019) raises a similar question:

> [H]ow are we to know which are the 'true' contradictions and which are the false? The theologian who makes do with the shop-worn old tools of classical logic and theology has a ready and easy answer: there are no 'true' contradictions.   (McCall, 2019)

This is clearly a fundamental question, a pressing one for the viability of Contradictory Christology.

Reply. Before addressing the fundamental epistemological question a clarification about true 'versus' false contradictions should be flagged.[13] For

---

[13] I should also note that I am unclear on why McCall uses scare quotes around 'true' in the context. My account is not that there's some special sense of 'true' – say, true* – whereby some contradictions are true*. My position is that some contradictions are true – full stop – in the usual sense of 'true'.

convenience, as throughout the book, let $!A$ be $A \wedge \neg A$ (with parentheses around it when necessary). On my account, reflected in the truth and falsity conditions for logical negation (and logical nullation, though this is logically redundant), any true contradiction is a false contradiction: $!A$ is true just if $\neg !A$ is true too. Put in terms of true theories, a true theory contains an application of logic's truth operator (viz., †) to a contradiction $!A$ just when it contains an application of logic's falsity operator (viz., $\neg$) to $!A$ too – that is, $†!A$ is in a true theory just when $\neg !A$ is in the true theory too. So, if we have a true contradiction, we thereby have a false contradiction too.

McCall's question, in light of the terminological clarification above, is really just this: which are the true contradictions? The answer, to the frustration of truth-seeking theorists everywhere, is the usual one: namely, *that's the question we're all trying to answer!*

Take a step back to the general question of which McCall's is a special instance: namely, which are the true sentences? If there were a simple answer to this question prior to arrival at the answer, our search for truth would be very much easier than it is – to put things mildly. Indeed, even if there were a complicated but largely algorithmic answer to this question, our search for truth would be vastly easier than it is. But such is not the way things are. Sorting the truths from the rest is a messy and very, very difficult business, one still nicely illustrated by the old Neurath–Quine metaphor of rebuilding our raft at sea (Quine, 1969). Accordingly, there is no simple answer to the general form of McCall's question – an answer which would sort all truths from the rest.

Of course, McCall's question is explicitly not the general one; it concerns only contradictions. And in that case – the case of contradictions – one might suggest that there ought to be a simple answer. But why? Consider the same question concerning 'ought' sentences: which of them are the true ones? Or 'it is necessary that . . .' sentences: which of them are the true ones? And so on for any form of sentence: which of them are true? Truth-seeking inquiry is complicated precisely because there simply isn't an easy answer to such questions.

But one might still press the particular example to which McCall points: namely, *contradictions*. As McCall rightly says, if we adopt the mainstream theory of logical consequence (viz., so-called classical logic) we get an easy answer to at least that question (of contradictions): namely, *none of 'em* – full stop. But getting an easy answer to the given question is not itself good reason to accept the easy-answer-giving theory. If it were, we'd have good reason to accept the trivial theory of every phenomenon.[14] After all, trivialism gives the easiest answer to figuring out the truths: namely, *all of 'em.*

McCall is correct that on my account logic does not help with respect to sorting truths of the form !*A* any more than logic helps with sorting truths of the dual form <*A* (where <*A* is ¬*A* ∨ *A*). In this respect, my account makes our epistemological situation with respect to such sentences appear to be more difficult than the standard account of logic affords. But if my account is correct, our epistemological situation was always just that difficult: it wasn't logic classifying !*A* as logically false or logic classifying <*A* as logically true; it was our extralogical theorizing, perhaps backed by various methodological practices (with respect to default rejection of !*A* and/or default acceptance of <*A*) that did the given epistemological work. For all that I can see, few if any of such practices are jeopardized by an account according to which there is a strikingly rare contradictory being.

But one might still press: if we accept the existence of even one contradictory being – regardless of how strikingly radical, strikingly bizarre, and strikingly abnormal the being appears to be – we are no longer justified in a default rejection of contradictory accounts of any other being.

That's incorrect. This book is not the place to take up such a huge epistemological issue. But let me reply as clearly and concisely as I can: such a charge is untrue. To put my epistemological cards on the table: I accept a rather crude form of so-called epistemic conservatism (Harman, 1986, 1999) according to which we are justified in what we accept unless we have some special reason to reject it. (This is the dual of a crude Cartesian foundationalism, according to which we are unjustified in what we accept unless we have some special reason to accept it.) For all that I can tell, the history of truth-seeking disciplines, aimed mostly at the normal diet of examples, has run smoothly and successfully on a default rejection of gluts (and likewise gaps). Things have not gone so well when it comes to the bizarre phenomena that appear to all reflective lights to be wildly paradoxical, paranormal, or otherwise beyond the standard run of examples. Such phenomena scream out against our normal – indeed, widely default – extra-logical practices of acceptance–rejection behavior. The default principles that guide our standard acceptance–rejection behavior are not jeopardized by being rendered inapplicable in some rare cases; they're just shown, to nobody's surprise, not

---

[14] The trivial theory in a language L is the theory containing all sentences of L.

to be more than standardly applicable – more than good, reliable but still only default principles.

4.2.3 What level of support is required?

McCall (2019) raises the following question:

> A second question is closely related to the first: what is the level of required support that is needed to establish the truth of both claims of a contradiction?   (McCall, 2019)

The question demands a response.

Reply. My reply to the question, as it stands, is straightforward: one needs the support that shows them to be true. What is that? Again, as in §4.2.2, the standards of truth are what they are; and the difficulties of our epistemic position with respect to finding truth are also what they are – typically, very difficult. The bar of truth does not discriminate among candidates: for a sentence – no matter what it is – to be true is, well, for it to be true. Put 'graphically', the truth of

'Snow is white' is true.

requires nothing more nor less than that snow is white. Likewise, the truth of

The consequence relation for metaphysical necessity is so-called S5.

requires nothing more nor less than that the true theory of metaphysical necessity (whatever that is) be closed under the so-called S5 consequence relation. Likewise, the truth of

It's false that Christ is mutable.

requires nothing more nor less than that it's false that Christ is mutable. And yet again, likewise, the truth of

It's true that Christ is mutable.

requires nothing more nor less than that it's true that Christ is mutable. And so on, including logical conjunctions of such claims. In particular, the truth of

It's false that Christ is mutable and it's true that Christ is mutable.

requires nothing more nor less than what is required for the truth of the respective conjuncts.

As stated, McCall's question is answered as above. But McCall is in fact after more, where the more is expressed in three more questions as follows (each taken verbatim from McCall 2019):

1. If two theological propositions taken together seem to produce a contradiction, does that give us reason to go back and look closely at the data or evidence (whether textual, empirical, experiential, or just what) supporting the propositions?
2. If another non-contradictory theory is not impossible and also makes more-or-less adequate sense of the data, is that one to enjoy a prefer-ence (at least initially)? If so, then why?
3. Just how much support for the propositions must one have to embrace something that surely is an actual contradiction?

As McCall says, 'at some point answers to such questions will be important if [Contradictory Christology] is to put down theological roots and produce some doctrinal fruit' (McCall, 2019).

By way of reply I offer the following as directions towards answers, not as fully developed answers to McCall's given questions.

Reply to (1): It depends on what 'seems' means here. Take the fundamental problem itself. Here, the central truths of Christ, as recorded in Chalcedon and creeds, screamingly seem to be contradictory – right on their surface, right from the get-go. And yet, even with their screaming contradictoriness, they stand as defining truth. Given the centrality of the apparent contradic-toriness of such (fundamental-problem) truths, going back to 'eke out' a non-contradictory substitute strikes me as misguided, or at least without good reason.[15] But if 'seems' in McCall's question flags that we are talking about

---

[15] The 'eke out' terminology is from Coakley (2002), quoted by McCall in a different dialectical context of his paper.

more tenuous, less central facets of theology than the apparent contradiction of Christ displayed on the very welcome sign of Chalcedon-constrained Christology, then following the normal default rejection of a contradictory conclusion is probably reasonable. (I say 'probably' because, of course, details really do matter in these sorts of *what-do-I-do-here* sort of question.) Again, the search for truth is hard no matter the area. Theology, as McCall reminds, is certainly no different. But the bar, as in §4.2.2, is the same throughout: the support required for the truth of A is, well, whatever is sufficient for A's truth. Unlike separating sheep from goats, there is no general recipe that one can follow to separate the truths from the untruths. There are simply general rules of epistemic responsibility, including *think carefully*; *be as unbiased as you can in the pursuit of truth*; *be open but not hoodwinked by inspiration* (e.g., revelation); and many other general (but imprecise) such rules.

Reply to (2): I take this question as follows. Suppose that we have a con-tradictory theory and a non-contradictory theory as theoretically possible candidates for the truth of a given phenomenon. (In other words, from our current epistemic position, the logical possibility of a glutty theory of the phenomenon is not ruled out.) Moreover, suppose that both candidates make equally good sense of the phenomenon (or the data concerning the phenomenon as the target of our theory). Does the non-contradictory theory enjoy some higher level of probability?

The answer to the question depends a little bit on the space of possibilities in question. If the space is equally (or even roughly equally) divided between glutty candidates and non-glutty candidates, the answer to the question is negative. If, on the other hand, the space has just a few glutty candidates compared with a vast multitude of non-glutty candidates, then the answer is affirmative. Pending details, there is not a lot more to say by way of answer.

Reply to (3): Even though (3) is answered in §4.2.2 it is worth repeating that we do seem to have a longstanding successful practice of rejecting logic's glutty possibilities as leading candidates for the truth of a phenomenon. The practice revolves around 'normal cases', things that offer up little suggestion of being glutty (or gappy). If, at bottom, McCall's epistemological questions are fueled by the practical question of whether we should continue the given default methodological practice with respect to gluts (and/or gaps), my reply is: yes. And if one asks whether the 'yes' here is defeasible the answer is: yes. After all, we are not only in a difficult epistemic situation with respect to finding truth; we are also epistemically fallible through and through.

The existence of true contradictions (gluts) neither helps nor hurts our epistemic predicament, as far as I can see. Those who, perhaps with McCall, think that the logical possibility of gluts (or gaps) wreaks havoc on our pursuit of truth are mistaken, as far as I can see. The chief effect of such logical possibilities is not havoc; the effect is simply that logic itself no longer explains our default practice of rejecting gluts (gaps). By my lights, this is not a negative effect.

4.2.4 Implausible

Accepting that Christ exemplified a property and its logical complement is downright implausible. As such the proposed Contradictory Christology is implausible.

Reply. If the objection is an empirical claim about what human believers can in fact believe then the objection needs to be evaluated empirically. But there are philosophers who in fact believe of various entities that they instantiate a property and the property's logical complement. Pending further empirical tests such philosophers appear to be counterexamples to the sort of empirical charge of implausibility advanced in the objection.

But perhaps 'implausible' is used in a weaker sense: it's *hard to believe*; it's *nearly incredible (nearly not believable)*, and so on. But in this case, such a property is to be expected of the true christology. After all, the true story of Christ – the true story of the extraordinary GodMan – is nearly beyond belief. That christian theologians of all stripes have emphasized the necessity of faith in the face of 'implausibility' or even 'foolishness' is not an objection to the truth; it's (at least in part) a recognition of the implausibility of the truth.

4.2.5 Which comes first: logic or consequence?

Cotnoir (2019) raises another epistemological question which is based on his characterization of my view. In characterizing my view of logic (-al consequence) Cotnoir puts matters thus:

> [A]ccording to Beall...logic [-al consequence] is common to all theory-relative entailment relations. That is, *an argument is logically valid if and only if the premises entail the conclusion according to every consequence*

relation. This last biconditional invites the following question: which determines which? What is the order of explanation? Is universal logic [i.e., *logic, logical consequence*] primary, and so determines the space of possible consequence relations? Or are theory-relative consequence relations primary, and logic is determined simply by looking at their intersections?

(Cotnoir, 2019)

Pending an answer, Contradictory Christology is saddled with, at best, a sorely partial – unhelpfully incomplete – account of logical consequence.

Reply. I have three comments by way of reply.

First comment. While the left–right direction of Cotnoir's biconditional is (in effect) true by definition of 'logic' (qua the consequence relation involved in those of all true theories) the converse (viz., right–left) direction is dubious unless it's supposed to be (for lack of a better term) 'true by redundancy'. The right–left direction says that if all claims in X jointly entail A according to every theory-specific consequence relation $\vdash_T$ in every true theory T, then all claims in X jointly entail A according to logic. In notation, where $\vdash$ (unsubscripted) is logical consequence and $\vdash_T$ the consequence (closure) relation for true theory T:

LT. If $X \vdash_T A$ for every true theory T, then $X \vdash A$.

LT is true if logic is among the $\vdash_T$ relations in the antecedent of LT; but if logic itself is not among the consequence relations talked about by LT's antecedent then I do not see any reason to accept LT. (There could be something very strange like a piece of vocabulary – maybe some identity relation – that happens to show up in all true theories but is not part of logical vocabulary, and so is not something on which logic itself makes a claim.) But now the issue: if Cotnoir's biconditional is true then its truth falls out of either redundancy (in the right–left direction) or, in effect, definition (in the left–right direction).

Second comment. Why think that there's an interesting order-of-explanation question if the biconditional is as above, namely, either true by redundancy or true by definition? I don't see it.

Third comment. Cotnoir's order-of-explanation question concerns the space of logic's possibilities versus that of narrower spaces invoked by many of our true theories (e.g., when they rule out glutty logical possibilities or gappy logical possibilities as theoretical impossibilities or just run-of-the-mill possibilities that are beyond what the theory recognizes as possible for its target phenomenon). In §2, among other places, I claim that logical space – the space of logic's possibilities – is the broadest space, and our true theories narrow the space of logic's possibilities to zero in on their respective spaces of theory-specific possibilities. But Cotnoir's question is epistemological (versus, say, ontological): which do we know first? On this question I have no useful answer. Like most epistemological questions, we remain at sea rebuilding our raft (to use a worn-out but still accurate metaphor). We do the best we can in pursuing the truth of things. If pressed, I don't think I could confidently even venture a guess. As far as I know, the search for true theories might fix a candidate for logical consequence while it pursues candidates for its target phenomenon (say, biology, or maths, or theology), only to sink and then surface again to hold fixed the candidate for theology (or maths, biology or whatever) while searching for the true theory of logic. Biological life for each of us seems to have an order from beginning to end, with roughly predictable stages in between those points; but the progression towards the discovery of true theories – true theories of anything, let alone everything – is anything but so ordered. If we knew in advance that we had the truth about logic's possibilities, we'd have a much easier epistemological life than we do. But we don't. Of course, on my view, if we know that we have the true theory about some phenomenon then we thereby know that we have at least a partial description of the true account of logic's possibilities. But as a general rule, judging between the epistemic chicken and the epistemic egg is not very fruitful. There is absolutely a truth of the matter; but I've no idea what it is, and I'm not sure that it matters a great deal to whether logic plays the role in theology (and other truth-seeking disciplines) that I say it does.

4.3 Theological issues

4.3.1 Heretical

Contradictory Christology is heretical in that the theory has heretical claims as consequences.[16]

---

[16] Dave Ripley pushed this objection at a UNAM Conference in Mexico. The objection is a more direct version of an objection by Anderson (2007, p. 125f), namely, Anderson's third (and, by his lights, weightiest) objection against a glut-theoretic theology. I treat the other two of Anderson's three objections in separate objections below; I discuss his version of the current objection in a long parenthetical remark (page 70).

You maintain that Christ's divine nature entails Christ's impassibility:

1. That Christ is divine entails that Christ is impassible.

(1), together with similar entailments, gives rise to the fundamental 'problem' of Christology. The trouble is that *entailment* contraposes, that is,

2. If *A* entails *B* then ¬*B* entails ¬*A*.

Hence, from (1) and (2), we have (3) as a consequence, namely:

3. That Christ is passible entails that Christ is not divine.

But, now, since the theory contains the claim that Christ is passible we get from (3) the heretical (4):

4. Christ is not divine.

This is plainly heretical. And the same argument goes through to show that Contradictory Christology, as you develop it, claims other heresies – such as that Christ is not human. Inasmuch as Contradictory Christology is supposed to be compatible with Chalcedon-constrained christology, the current objection shows that Contradictory Christology fails, and should therefore be rejected.

** *Long parenthetical remark.* As above, an objection by James Anderson, which is of a kind with the current objection, is that Contradictory Christology winds up making the preservation of orthodoxy irrelevant because it is (allegedly) forced to make heretical claims (Anderson, 2007, p. 125f). Anderson's exact objection points to identity claims that, he alleges, would arise from a glutty approach to the trinity (about which I've said nothing here, but say something about in §6). By my lights this is a bad example; it's a hard task for any theory to come up with the right identity relation, and perhaps especially so for christian theology, and especially as involving doctrines of the trinity. But one thing is pretty clear: either identity in christian theology (especially the relation involved in the trinity) will not be transitive or it will invalidate the sort of substitution principles on which Anderson's objection relies. Anderson just assumes that either it is transitive or it allows for familiar substitution (or both). He might be thinking that logic itself has an identity predicate, and so, inasmuch as logical vocabulary is universal and part of every theory, that predicate is involved in christian theology. That logic has an identity predicate is incorrect, as I see things; logic does not have an identity predicate (identity relations are not topic-neutral enough to be logical), and even if it did it would hardly be even an equivalence relation. Moreover, even if, contrary to what I think is the correct account, logic had an identity predicate there's no reason to think that that predicate is the one involved in expressing the axiomatic truths of the trinity. Furthermore, even if the correct account of the trinity – and in particular trinitarian identity – should ultimately be glut-theoretic, and if it should ultimately appear to contain heretical claims, an important distinction between different 'forms of heresy' needs to be drawn, and with it, Anderson's given objection is not strong by my lights. (On the relevant 'forms of heresy' see the distinction between H1 and H2, defined below, page 71.) *End remark.* **

Reply. There are two important parts of the reply.

The first part of the reply is to note that heresies need to be understood in a way compatible with the possibility of Contradictory Christology. In particular, a familiar heresy concerning Christ's divinity may be understood in at least two ways:

H1. *Presence of Negation:* the theory contains the given negation (viz., 'It's false that Christ is divine').

H2. *Absence of Nullation:* the theory fails to contain the given 'nullation' (viz., 'It is true that Christ is divine').

The current objection charges that Contradictory Christology, as advanced here, commits a heresy in the H1 sense; but there is no suggestion that the theory commits a heresy in the H2 sense. By my lights, it would not be surprising were the truth of Christ, who is the unique contradictory being at the center of christian theology, to involve 'heresies' in the H1 sense. After all, that Christ exemplifies two complementary natures (the joint satisfaction of which entails a contradiction) may bring about falsity claims that appear to be deeply heretical (i.e., H1-heretical); but the substantial heresies, at least by my lights, involve an outright rejection of the orthodox claims – the absence of such claims from our christology. The substance of serious heresy is in H2: namely, having a theory that omits the given truth (e.g., that Christ is divine, that Christ is human, etc.).

The second part of the reply is to refute the claim that Contradictory Christology, as advanced here, commits a heresy even in the H1 sense. What the objection assumes is that our christology's consequence relation – our entailment relation for our theory of Christ – contraposes. This assumption is erroneous. Indeed, the objection illustrates precisely why the entailment relation for true christology fails to contrapose.

It is true that *logical* entailment (viz., FDE, as outlined above) contraposes: if the entailment relation in premise (2) of the objection concerns only logical entailment, then premise (2) is correct. But if premise (2) is talking about logical entailment, then – for the objection's argument to work – premise (1) is also talking about logical entailment. But (1) should be rejected if it is talking about logical entailment, since logic is completely neutral on things like possibility and human natures; such things are beyond the sparse, topic-neutral logical vocabulary. If (1) is true – and it is true – then (1) is not talking about logical entailment; it's talking about the entailment (or consequence) relation involved in our specific theological theory. And there's no reason to think that that relation contraposes. (Indeed, as above, there's reason – in the objection – to think that it doesn't.)

The foregoing reply answers the objection; however, the point is critical to the overall position, and any lingering unclarity needs to be removed. Indeed, Pawl (2019a) highlights some remaining questions around my claim that theological consequence (i.e., true theology's consequence relation) doesn't contrapose even though logical consequence – which is universal and involved in the consequence relations of all true theories – does contrapose. Pawl writes:[17]

> ... [You say] that the correct Christology-specific consequence relation does not contrapose.... I'm not sure how this works. [You also] say that 'It is true that *logical* entailment ... contraposes' ... and that 'logical consequence governs *all cases whatsoever*; logic is topic-neutral, universal, and is not at all subject to a particular corner of reality'.... [You] also [say] ... that logical consequence 'is part of *every* consequence relation involved in any of our theories'.... [Following italics mine:] *So, it looks to me as if logical*

[17] Here, I thread Pawl's initial main-body text with his footnote 7 in which his concern arises (Pawl, 2019a, fn. 7). Pawl's given paper is very clear that the following issue is not directly related to Pawl's principal dialectical aims, which is why he puts the highlighted unclarity in a footnote. But, again, the unclarity that Pawl highlights is important to address even if only ancillary to his direct dialectical aims.

consequence is part of the consequence relation of theology. But then since logical consequence contraposes, it looks to me as if the theology-specific consequence relation should contrapose too, contra what [you say].

(Pawl, 2019a)

The italicized part at the end is the center of the unclarity. Clarity is achieved by clarifying the sense in which logical consequence is part of theology's (and every true theory's) consequence relation.

Let $\vdash$ (unsubscripted) be logical consequence and let $\vdash_\Theta$ be theological consequence (*Theta* for theological consequence). In turn, read '$X \vdash A$' as 'X logically entails A' and likewise, mutatis mutandis, for '$X \vdash_\Theta A$'. (Here, X is either a set of sentences or, for simplicity for present purposes, just one sentence.) Now, logic is part of theology's consequence relation in that the latter 'extends' the former:

- Theological consequence (viz., $\vdash_\Theta$) *extends* logical consequence (viz., $\vdash$) iff if $X \vdash A$ then so too $X \vdash_\Theta A$.

There's nothing peculiar about theological consequence; every true theory has a consequence relation that extends logic (in the sense above). And in that sense, logical consequence is 'universal' – it's part of every true theory's consequence relation. If $X \therefore A$ is valid according to logic (i.e., logically valid) then $X \therefore A$ is T-valid for every true theory T, including the true theology. That's all there is to logic's being a part of every true theory's consequence relation: namely, the theory's consequence relation 'obeys' logic on any 'form' that logic declares to be valid.

Importantly, what is not involved in logic's given universality (i.e., in its being a part of every consequence relation involved in every true theory) is that for every true theory T, anything true of logical consequence is thereby true of T-consequence. In particular, what is not involved in logic's universality is that anything true of logical consequence is thereby true of $\vdash_\Theta$, true theology's consequence relation. But that's where Pawl's highlighted unclarity persists. In particular, logical consequence contraposes: if A logically entails B, then $\neg B$ logically entails $\neg A$. (In notation above: if $A \vdash B$ then $\neg B \vdash \neg A$.) But this doesn't entail that every consequence relation that extends logical consequence contraposes; and in particular, according to me, theological consequence doesn't contrapose.

There are two ways to diminish the unclarity around this point. The first route: what argument would establish that $\vdash_\Theta$ contraposes if $\vdash$ (logic) does?[18] The second route: is there a simple counterexample? I'll briefly address each route in turn.

4.3.1.1 Argument for target contraposition?

In highlighting the target unclarity Pawl's discussion gestures at an argument from logic's contraposing to the contraposition of theological consequence. The argument seems to be as follows, where '$A \vdash B$' and '$A \vdash_\Theta B$' express that A logically entails B and, respectively, that A theologically entails B.

1. Fact: if $A \vdash B$ then $A \vdash_\Theta B$. [Logic is part of $\vdash_\Theta$.]
2. Fact: if $A \vdash B$ then $\neg B \vdash \neg A$. [Logic contraposes.]
3. * *Suppose*: $A \vdash B$.
4. * $\neg B \vdash \neg A$. [2, 3]
5. * $\neg B \vdash_\Theta \neg A$. [1,4]
6. *Hence*: if $A \vdash B$ then $\neg B \vdash_\Theta \neg A$. [3,4,5]

Is there anything wrong with this argument? No; the argument is sound.[19] But one must be clear about what the argument does (not) establish.

The argument *does* establish its conclusion: namely, that if logic declares that $A \therefore B$ is valid then theological consequence declares $\neg B \therefore \neg A$ to be valid – in short, that if $A \vdash B$ then $\neg B \vdash_\Theta \neg A$. (The same holds for every consequence relation involved in any of our true theories.) But this fact is not the one towards which Pawl's argument is directed.

The argument above is sound but does *not* establish Pawl's key desideratum, namely, that theological consequence itself contraposes: namely,

- $\vdash_\Theta$ contraposition: if $A \vdash_\Theta B$ then $\neg B \vdash_\Theta \neg A$.

In that respect, the argument is defective; it misses its target.

4.3.1.2 Counterexample to target contraposition?

The search for a sound argument from the contraposition of logic to the contraposition of theological consequence is not fruitful; in fact, it is doomed. There are counterexamples that refute the would-be target. One counterexample, from my view, is made plain in the fallacious (because

---

[18] Generalizing, the issue seeks an argument for $\vdash_T$'s contraposing if $\vdash_*$ contraposes and $\vdash_T$ extends $\vdash_*$; but I'll focus on the particular case of logic and theology.

[19] Some readers might worry about the use of conditional proof here or even detachment from these conditionals; the worry is fully answered by the fact that this argument is done in the language of a (meta-) theory which validates such things.

equivocating) argument towards heresy discussed above. But there is a simpler though more abstract way to see how counterexamples emerge.

Here's one clear way to see how logic can contrapose but, even though $\vdash_\Theta$ (viz., theological consequence) never disobeys logic when logic claims that some pattern $X \therefore A$ is valid, $\vdash_\Theta$ itself doesn't contrapose. Let's suppose (not implausibly) that fundamental-problem properties – tied essentially to one of Christ's two natures – are truly (and/or falsely) exemplified by Christ in all of the possibilities recognized by the true theology. Take

1. Christ is immutable.

as an example. This, then, is true in all of theology's possibilities but, according to Contradictory Christology, likewise is false across all such possibilities; (1) is glutty in all models of the true theological theory. (This is what we're stipulating for the example.)

Notice that theology thereby carves out a proper part of the logical space of possibilities wherein there is a 'necessary glut', recognized as such by theology's consequence relation $\vdash_\Theta$. But this has direct effects on contraposition. To see this, let γ (gamma as heuristic for glut) be one of theology's necessary gluts: it is true and false at all models of the true theology, so that $\dagger\gamma$ (logic's truth operator applied to γ) and $\neg\gamma$ (logic's falsity operator applied to γ) are each true and false at all possibilities seen by theology's consequence relation. But, then, since γ is at least true at all possibilities seen by $\vdash_\Theta$, we have the following theology-valid form/pattern:

$$A \therefore \gamma$$

That is: $A \vdash_\Theta \gamma$. But now contrapose to get the form/pattern:

$$\neg\gamma \therefore \neg A$$

Since γ is glutty everywhere that $\vdash_\Theta$ sees, it's at least true every such where. But there are many sentences A in the language of theology that are just true (not also false) at many possibilities. All we need is one such A and one such possibility where A is just true; for at that possibility $\neg A$ is thereby just false, even though, as above, $\neg\gamma$ is glutty (and thereby at least true). Accordingly,

$$\neg\gamma \nvdash_\Theta \neg A$$

which is to say that $\neg\gamma$ does not theology-entail $\neg A$.

Putting the pieces of the example together, one can see that one (among other) ways that contraposition for $\vdash_\Theta$ fails arises from special features of the language of the theory (i.e., of theology) and in particular constraints on the space of theoretical possibilities that result in making some sentences necessarily glutty.[20]

But necessary gluts (or gaps) are not necessary for ruining contraposition in a theory's consequence relation. Suppose that, as some have suggested (in conversation), the true theology is a glut-only theology, treating logic's gappy possibilities as theoretical impossibilities.[21] Suppose, too, that there are no theoretically necessary gluts; it's just that the space of theoretical possibilities is exhausted by ones where sentences are either just true, just false, or they are glutty. (No gaps, though it's worth noting that the example can be run with no gluts and just gaps too.) In that case, even though (we're stipulating) there are no theoretically necessary gluts, theology's consequence relation fails to contrapose, largely for the same reason given above. To see this, note that without gaps in the picture the following is a true theological-entailment claim according to the given theological consequence relation:

$$A \vdash_\Theta B \vee \neg B$$

(Recall that FDE governs the truth and falsity conditions of the logical vocabulary; and so, without gaps, $B \vee \neg B$ cannot be made untrue; it is either just-true or it is a glut.) But now consider the contraposition:

$$\neg(B \vee \neg B) \therefore \neg A$$

This is not Θ-valid, that is,

$$\neg(B \vee \neg B) \nvdash_\Theta \neg A$$

To see this, go to a possibility, recognized by $\vdash_\Theta$, whereat A is just-true and B is a glut. As a walk through the truth/falsity conditions for logical negation

[20] Another route towards the same point points to theology-necessary gaps (if there are any), which are possible according to logic but which I've set aside as not directly relevant to Pawl's overall discussion.

[21] Mike Rea, Tim Pawl, Natalja Deng, and Gill Russell have independently suggested that a contradictory theology that is uniformly glutty or, dually, uniformly gappy enjoys a theoretical unity (and thereby some degree of theoretical attractiveness) over one that treats some theological 'problems' as gluts and some as 'gaps'. This sort of issue might motivate a glut-only theology approach to the trinity, which I tentatively discuss in §6.

and disjunction will reveal, $\neg(B \vee \neg B)$ is glutty in the given possibility too. But, then, $\neg(B \vee \neg B)$ can be (at least) true while $\neg A$ can be untrue – not even at least true. So, in light of the Θ-recognized counterexample, the given form is Θ-invalid, even though logic itself (viz., FDE) contraposes.

4.3.2   Awkward theological consequence

James Anderson (2007) gives various objections to a would-be glutty theology (i.e., a theology with at least 'truth-value gluts' about God).[22] The first is crisp and powerful:

> [Contradictory Christology] has the odd consequence that God believes some falsehoods (about God, no less) and invites us to do likewise. This criticism may not be decisive, but it seems hard to reconcile this outcome with the biblical emphasis on promoting truth and eschewing untruth (e.g., Ps. 52:3; Eph. 4:25; 1 John 4:6).   (Anderson, 2007, p. 125)

If Anderson is right then Contradictory Christology is both awkward and, more problematic, goes against Scripture.

Reply. The objection is not only not decisive; it simply repeats the core thesis of Contradictory Christology, namely, that the full truth of Christ involves falsehoods. If by 'odd consequence' is meant a surprising, unfamiliar, and strange consequence, then I am in agreement with the claim that Contradictory Christology has the given odd consequence. But this is not an objection. After all, all theologians agree that Christ's very being is surprising, unfamiliar, and very strange – if shown by nothing else than the fundamental problem of Christ's being.

---

[22] Anderson uses the now-not-uncommon term 'dialetheism' (sometimes 'dialethism', with adjective 'dialetheic' or 'dialethic') for any glut theory – that is, a theory that contains gluts (i.e., true falsehoods). Instead of that terminology I mostly use 'Contradictory Christology' to make Anderson's objection specific to my proposal.

On broader terminology: I prefer the simpler terminology of 'glut theory' (with adjective 'glutty'), which is the dual of 'gap theory' (with adjective 'gappy'); this simpler terminology predates the neologism 'dialetheism'. (Some glut theorists – including Graham Priest and Richard Sylvan (née Routley) who coined the term 'dialetheism' ('dialethism') – prefer the later terminology because they think that 'glut' carries negative connotations. I do not share such a view.) The original terminology of 'gluts' comes from Fine (1975).

God is omniscient. God knows the full truth of Christ. Since the full truth of Christ involves falsehoods (e.g., 'Christ is mutable', etc.) then some of God's knowledge is knowledge of falsehoods – which, of course, are also truths (since knowledge demands truth). True falsehoods are so rare as to make them strange, surprising, and very unfamiliar; and their existence comes about only in the strangest, most surprising cases – such as Christ.

Does this position go against Scripture's promotion of seeking truth and avoiding falsehood? No. Seeking truth is paramount; and falsehood is to be avoided at all costs short of losing truth. Scripture's dictate concerns the normal situation wherein truth and falsity are not inextricably bound together as they are in the unique case of Christ. In the case of Christ we pursue the full truth; and with it we wind up with falsehoods which are also true. Such is Christ's unique being.[23]

4.3.3 Phenomenological support

Anderson (2007) gives another objection to Contradictory Christology (and glutty theology generally), one that he takes to be as 'weighty' as the first (viz., his §4.3.2 above):

> [T]he law of non-contradiction enjoys considerable *prima facie* support by way of the phenomenology and ubiquity of belief in it. If nothing else, this indicates that a rejection of the law should serve only as a last resort in attempting to address the [fundamental problem]. Moreover, [a glutty] solution is likely to endear itself only to those standing *within* the Christian faith (and even then will be deemed a bitter pill). As a defensive strategy to counter the charge of irrationality levelled at Christian doctrines, it lacks plausibility and smacks of special pleading.   (Anderson, 2007, p. 125)

Reply. There are (again) many things that can be said by way of reply. I limit the reply to comments on four strands of the objection: 'the law of non-contradiction', the relevance of phenomenology to logic, the apparent ubiquity of said 'law', and the issue of defending christian theory against charges of irrationality.

---

[23] Also – lest there by any doubt – it's worth noting that the Scriptural texts that Anderson's objection highlight concern lying and deception (versus falsity on its own); and there is no part of Contradictory Christology that advocates lying or deception.

4.3.3.1 Non-contradiction

The term 'the law of non-contradiction' is notoriously ambiguous, as the philosophy of logic has made plain (e.g., Priest *et al.* 2004). On one hand, one might think that the law is a logically true sentence, something like *the logical conjunction of a sentence and its logical negation is false*, which is standardly symbolized

$$\neg(A \wedge \neg A)$$

where *A* is any sentence in the language of one's theory. But to express the logical truth of such a thing one uses the logical consequence relation (here symbolized as a single turnstile), namely:

$$\vdash \neg(A \wedge \neg A)$$

This is a top candidate for 'the' law of non-contradiction, but this can't be what Anderson (or others) have in mind, since this is compatible with glut theory.[24]

Another candidate is some sort of extra-logical principle about rational acceptance and rejection, namely, *that one ought (rationally) to reject all contradictions*, where a contradiction, as throughout, is the logical conjunction of a sentence and its logical negation. Of course, this is an exceedingly difficult principle to justify in the face of viable glut theories, especially if some of those glut theories are true – such as, as I have suggested, Contradictory Christology. At the very least, this sort of 'law of non-contradiction' – which concerns the thorny area of rational 'change in view' (Beall, 2015; Harman, 1986) – is question-begging if launched against the viability of Contradictory Christology. This too is not what I think is the central notion of non-contradiction.

The core notion of non-contradiction at issue for Contradictory Christology is a version that is directly incompatible with Contradictory Christology. This version of non-contradiction, on which I henceforth take the current objection to focus, is sometimes called 'ex contradictione quodlibet' or, with more flair, 'explosion' (the latter colorfully indicating that a jot of negation inconsistency explodes a theory into the absurd trivial theory, which is the

---

[24] The scheme is not logically true in FDE, which I take to be the right account of logic; however, even if it were logically true, as it is in a well-known extension of FDE called 'LP' (Asenjo, 1966; Priest, 1979), its logical truth wouldn't rule out the logical possibility of $A \wedge \neg A$ also being true for some *A*.

theory that contains all sentences of the language of the theory):

$$A, \neg A \vdash B$$

where A and B are any sentences of the given language, and $\vdash$ is logical consequence (and, hence, is part of *every* consequence relation involved in any of our theories). In what follows I shall take the objection to concern this 'law' – better described as a 'rule' – of non-contradiction: namely, that arbitrary A together with its logical negation $\neg A$ (and, hence, by logic, the contradiction $A \wedge \neg A$) logically entails B. Contradictory Christology rejects this 'law', and must do so on pain of a simply absurd christology – the trivial christology.

4.3.3.2 Phenomenology of explosion

The objection alleges that there is strong phenomenological support for non-contradiction. I question whether this is true. (Does it 'feel right' that 'Satan is a Christian' logically follows from the claim that Christ is passible and impassible – or, more explicitly, that Christ is passible and yet Christ is not passible?) Even if the phenomenological feel supports explosion as a logical principle, the methodology of following phenomenology in this context is unmotivated. After all, logical consequence governs *all cases whatsoever*; logic is topic-neutral, universal, and is not at all subject to a particular corner of reality. But phenomenology is notorious for being a product of parochial diets: your 'phenomenological feel' depends on what you've eaten (so to speak). Indeed, that non-contradiction, understood as above (viz., explosion), is entrenched in a standard account of logic (viz., so-called classical logic) is not surprising; the standard account of logic was built exclusively on the diet of (classical) mathematics – a key topic for philosophical reflection. But phenomena like vagueness, semantic or 'logical' paradoxes, let alone phenomena like the unique and unparalleled Christ, were not even on the table when the standard account was crafted. Trusting phenomenology to determine logical consequence is not a reliable strategy.

4.3.3.3 Apparent ubiquity of 'explosion'

The objection points out that explosion (as the relevant 'law' of non-contradiction) is apparently ubiquitous in our best theories. (The objection talks about 'ubiquity of belief in it', but it is clearer to talk in this context of its role in our best theories – which, presumably, reflect our beliefs, etc.) On this point the objection is clearly right: explosion looks to play a dominant role in many – perhaps most – of our theories. So, how do we explain the apparent ubiquity of explosion in our theories if explosion is to be rejected?

Here, we need (as always) to distinguish logical consequence (represented as the bare single turnstile above) from a given theory's consequence relation. Explosion, as a *logical* rule (using logical consequence), is rejected by all viable glut theories, and certainly by Contradictory Christology. But this does not mean that our theory-specific consequence relations do not exhibit explosion.

The topic is too big for this chapter but the point, in short, is simply that theory-specific consequence relations (say, $\vdash_T$, for some theory T), while building on top of logic (and so not transgressing logic in any way), often build a form of explosion into the theory. For example, in our true theory of arithmetic, logic itself (qua FDE, as above) does not demand explosion; it says that it's logically invalid. But arithmetic's consequence relation $\vdash_T$ builds in explosion by narrowing the class of logical possibilities down to the ones that the theory takes to be (theoretically) possible. In particular, the theory (unlike logic) rules out the possibility of gluts for any predicates involved in arithmetic by enforcing this condition:

$$\exists x(Fx \wedge \neg Fx) \vdash_T \perp$$

where '$\exists x$' stands for logic's 'there exists at least one x such that' and 'Fx' is an open sentence ('property' or predicate) of the language of arithmetic, and $\perp$ is a sentence that entails, according to the theory's consequence relation, all sentences of the theory.[25] The effect of this condition is to narrow the set of *theoretical possibilities* down to exactly two sorts: the trivial one (where everything is true) and non-glutty ones (ones where no contradiction is true). With such a restriction on every predicate in the language of the theory one can show that any model of the theory is either trivial or negation-consistent – which is all that classical-logic theories can achieve.

While there is a lot more that can be said on the ubiquity of 'explosion' in many of our best theories, this is not the place; however, enough has been said to indicate that the apparent (and, I agree, genuine) ubiquity of explosive consequence relations is compatible with the failure of explosion in logic and, in particular, in Christology.[26]

---

[25] I use a unary predicate for simplicity; the generalization to any finite arity is straightforward.

[26] For a lot more on how explosive consequence relations play important roles in our theories despite logic's failure to be explosive, see work on 'shrieking' (Beall, 2013a,c, 2015).

4.3.3.4 Defending christian theory against charges of irrationality

The objection points out that if the aim of a solution to the fundamental problem is to defend christian theology against the charge of irrationality (which is James Anderson's key aim in his given book) then Contradictory Christology – or any other glut-theoretic theology – is not likely to be a front-running candidate, since the charge of irrationality is likely to come from those who assume (erroneously) that rationality demands non-contradictory theories.

The objection, as I see things (and as covered in §4.5.1), is irrelevant to the truth of Contradictory Christology. The aim of christology is to give the truth of Christ. The heart of Contradictory Christology is that the truth of Christ is contradictory. If one charges that *that* – the contradiction – is irrational, then let the objector state her grounds for saying as much. I have little doubt that the objector's 'grounds' will ultimately point to the standard account of logic, and also point to principles tying the given account of logic to (a theory of) rational acceptance–rejection behavior. While these are difficult matters to adjudicate, there is enough work in the philosophy of logic (and theories of rational acceptance–rejection behavior) to question the strength of such legs in the objector's charge.

Let me be perfectly plain: my aim is not to win debate; my aim is to get at the truth. And when it comes down to it, I find it very difficult to see how the standard account of logic can be the right account given the existence of bizarre phenomena like Christ – or of much lesser, theology-independent entities like common paradoxical phenomena. But if logic itself doesn't rule out the gluttiness of such entities then an argument is required for the view that something else does. Pending such an argument, I conclude that the objection remains irrelevant to the truth of Contradictory Christology, or some related contradictory theology in general.

4.3.4 True theology 'versus' other true theories?

Cotnoir (2019, §3.3) suggests that God's transcendence puts the true theology in a different category from other true theories – a difference in kind, not just status. If Cotnoir is correct in this claim then Contradictory Christology – and any logic-bound christology or theology – is at best fruitless.

Reply. Cotnoir's claim rests on two different lines of argument to suggest that the true theology is different in kind from other true theories. *The first line* points to a human–divine difference:

> Recall that logic is primarily delineated by a set of expressions — 'and', 'or', 'not', etc. — the logical vocabulary. But these expressions are directly tied to human natural language. " [T]he target always remains on 'real logical consequence' for our 'real language' " [Beall, 'Christ – A Contradiction']. Logic is, for Beall, fundamentally human.   (Cotnoir, 2019)

This is ambiguous. Logic, *as a human activity*, is human. That's true. But logic, *as an activity* (e.g., coming up with an account of logical consequence), is not necessarily a human activity; any entity capable of theorizing about logical consequence can engage in the activity. But set the *activity* of logic (of theorizing about logical consequence) aside. The more important disambiguation of Cotnoir's claim concerns logic *qua relation on all true theories*. There's nothing 'fundamentally human' about that relation. Sure, we, as humans, have used our language(s) to express what we take to be the true theory of logical consequence; but that makes logical consequence no more a fundamentally human relation than our true theory of arithmetic makes the number 2 or the successor function fundamentally human objects.

Disambiguated, Cotnoir is right that when we are doing logic – coming up with what we take to be the true account of logical consequence – we are humans who are engaged in a human activity (though the activity is not necessarily restricted to humans); however, Cotnoir is wrong to suggest that there's something 'fundamentally human' about the object of our true theory of logical consequence. The fact that logical consequence governs our many human languages, and governs the fragments that serve as languages of our many true theories, does not make logical consequence somehow relative to those languages. The language of the true logic (i.e., true theory of logical consequence) expresses the truth about logical consequence; but similarly the language of true biology expresses the truth about salamanders – and we shouldn't conclude that salamanders are fundamentally human.

Cotnoir's first line of argument for the view that true theology is importantly different from other true theories turns on a fallacious step from theology's expression in a human language to the objects of the theology being tied to the human mind or language or theory. This, I've argued above, is insufficient to show an important difference between theological theories and non-theological theories.

Cotnoir's *second line of argument* points not to the medium in which the theory is expressed but at the target phenomenon of the theory. In particular, Cotnoir argues that the transcendence of God (a feature of God which, I note, we can truly express just so) places theological theories in a different kind of category from non-theological ones. Cotnoir writes:

> There's a fundamental disanaology ... between theology and other human theorizing. When we seek out an appropriate consequencce relation for other target phenomena, we don't antecedently assume that the object of that inquiry transcends our conceptual scheme in important ways. Nor do we have to grapple with the possibility that the target's perfectly accurate self-understanding may be at odds with our own best theory.
>
> (Cotnoir, 2019)

Cotnoir is herein talking about theorizing – as an activity – and not obviously theories. I have no disagreement with the view that theological theorizing is different from other sorts of truth-seeking theorizing inasmuch as God (viz., the object of the theorizing) is supposed to be beyond a complete description in our finite theories. This puts the theorizer in a different place from other phenomena which may turn out to defy complete descriptions but are generally not themselves the creator of such limits. So, of course, there are these epistemological and in some ways psychological differences between theological theorizing and theorizing about other things. True, but how does that result in an important difference in kind from the resulting theories? I don't see it.

Where Cotnoir's argument is supposed to reach is that the role of logic in theology is different from the role of logic in other theories; and so there's a resulting difference (in kind) between the given sorts of theories. But nothing that Cotnoir has argued supports as much. Any argument from

» the object of our theory — namely, God — is fundamentally supposed to be (i.e., axiomatized to be) transcendent

to

» the role of logic in the theory is (thereby) different from all other theories is fallacious. After all, we still do our best to give as complete and true a theory of said object as possible—unless, of course, the true theory is that there can be no true theory of said object, which, I take it, is no part whatsoever of what the given argument is supposed to entail (and no part whatsoever of what Cotnoir himself aims to advance).[27]

In the end, there are differences between theological theorizing and non-theological theorizing; Cotnoir has not provided good reason to think that the true theology is different in kind from other true theories, and in particular different in the role that logic plays in such theories.

4.3.5 Theological explosion

Pawl (2019a) claims that even if – as I hold – logic doesn't validate the explosion of (formal) contradictions (i.e., even if there is no *logical* entailment from the logical conjunction of an arbitrary sentence and its logical negation to any arbitrary sentence) Contradictory Christology, as I advance it, is still not viable because explosions of contradictions (i.e., entailments from contradictions to all sentences in the language of the theory) come from quarters other than logic. This is a fundamental claim, reaching to the very roots of any would-be contradictory christology – and any would-be contradictory christian theology generally.

Reply. Pawl's given claim can be viewed as a dilemma: either Contradictory Christology entails the trivial theology or it results in a trivial scientific theory. Put just so, Pawl's dilemma looks like nothing more than a question-begging one; but it's not – at all. Pawl gives two arguments for his given claim, one (for the first horn) concerning the salient practice of theologians in the face of contradictions, the other concerning cross-disciplinary – inter-theoretical – truths common to both theology and (in his example) biology. If either of the two supporting arguments is successful, then Contradictory Christology – and, generally, any contradictory theology – should be rejected. But neither of Pawl's given arguments supports his principal claim, as I argue below.

---

[27] Even those like Eschenauer Chow (2018), who think that our true theories of God are at best analogically true, will reject that there's no true theory of a transcendent God.

Throughout his discussion, so as not to beg the question against Contradictory Christology, Pawl grants – for discussion – that logical consequence (i.e., logic itself) recognizes the possibility of gluts (true contradictions), and hence that logic itself doesn't treat contradictions as explosive sentences. While logic doesn't demand that true theories treat contradictions as explosive sentences (nor does it demand that they don't), many true theories rule out the logical possibility of gluts (true contradictions) by treating them as theoretical impossibilities. It is just such theory-specific 'explosion' from contradictions that Pawl's principal objection concerns. His first horn is the claim that true theology itself rules out gluts as theoretically impossible.

4.3.5.1 From theological practice?
Pawl's argument for the claim that contradictions are explosive sentences in true theology points to theological practice itself. Why point to theological practice? Pawl does this in response to a prior question in the face of logic's treating contradictions one way (viz., as not explosive sentences) and yet many other consequence relations involved in our true theories treating them differently (viz., as explosive). Pawl puts matters this way:

> Here's a question at this junction: how do we determine which theory-specific consequence relations preclude true contradictions or build in explosion, and which do not? Whatever our answer to that question is, it shouldn't require us to become experts in every theory to check for ourselves whether it requires explosion. Rather, we should trust the judgement of the expert theorists.   (p. 7)

There seem to be two questions here:

Q1. How do we tell whether a theory's consequence relation validates explosion for contradictions (i.e., validates the entailment from arbitrary contradiction !A to arbitrary sentence B)?

Q2. How do we determine whether theorists implicitly assume that the true theory of their theory's consequence relation – whenever it is explicitly recorded – validates explosion for contradictions?

Q1 has an easy-to-state answer: we look at the true theory of the given theory's consequence relation. Such a theory will tell us whether the given consequence relation validates explosion for contradictions. Pawl assumes (correctly, I think) that theologians have not formulated the true theory of theology's consequence relation, at least not in full; and so Pawl's pointing to theological practice is intended to answer not Q1 but Q2, and do so in the affirmative:

> By my lights, the overwhelming majority of theologians employ inference rules that would preclude true contradictions in their theological work.
>
> (p. 7)

I agree with Pawl on this: namely, that theologians seem to work on the assumption that contradictions are explosive – that they are not in the space of theological possibilities. But that's not the important question.

We're assuming – Pawl is conceding (at least for debate) – that logic itself doesn't underwrite the given assumption of 'the overwhelming majority'. The pressing question, then, is: why – in the face of the apparent contradiction of Christ – should theologians rule out the possibility of gluts? Why, in the face of the central apparent contradiction, should theologians assume that the consequence relation in true theology validates explosion for contradictions? It is this question to which 'expert opinion' is directly relevant – and directly required.

Pawl explicitly discusses the work of Gabriel Biel.[28] Biel is plainly aware of the apparent contradiction of Christ (i.e., aware of 'the fundamental problem'). His solution to the fundamental problem, a predecessor of Pawl's own, rejects the standard satisfaction conditions of predicates like 'mutable' and 'immutable' (etc.) in favor of a non-standard usage (explained at length in Pawl's 2016 monograph on conciliar christology). Why reject the standard usage? Biel's answer (as quoted by Pawl p. 7) is plain:

> ...because [the standard conditions] imply contradictories of the same thing   [viz., Christ].

My response: right, that's the apparent contradiction of Christ; and that's the fundamental problem at issue. But the question is: why reject that the apparent contradiction of Christ is veridical? Why reject that there are contradictories true of Christ?

Biel simply doesn't answer the question, at least not as far as I know. The first-cab-off-the-block answer, of course, is that Biel rejects the possibility of a

---

[28] For scholarship on Biel see Cross 2019.

contradictory Christ – indeed, a contradictory anything – because *logic* itself rules out such 'possibilities'. My conjecture is that that's the answer that Biel would give were anyone to actually put the current question to him: namely, that logic rules out such a 'possibility', and hence our true theory of Christ – and true theology generally – has no such 'possibility' to entertain. Whether Biel would say as much is something I leave to experts in Biel's work. For present purposes, saying as much is unavailable; for, as above, Pawl assumes (at least for debate) that logic itself does not rule out the possibility of gluts – does not rule out an entity of which/whom contradictories are true.

What, then, for present purposes, is the lesson we should draw from Biel's plain and firm rejection of contradictions in theology – and, indeed, from the vast majority of theologians whose careful work reflects a rejection of gluts in theology? Pending explicit discussion of their reasons for doing so, I do not see a clearly relevant lesson to draw (i.e., relevant to the issue of whether the true theology rules out gluts). The widespread rejection of gluts in theology is not itself good reason to think that the true theology is glut-free.

The need for some account of why contradictions are taken to be explosive in theology is especially pressing given the historical and conceptual oddity of the central fact in the christian worldview: namely, the incarnation of God – the walking, talking union of 'transcendence and immanence' – who is not many but one person, 'fully divine' and 'fully human', with all that those natures entail. To many a sympathetic mind, even within committed realms of traditional monotheism, such an alleged fact appears to be nonsense, its nonsensicality falling freely from its prima facie logical impossibility. Of course, if true contradictions really were logically impossible, then mainstream theological practice would be right to sing as much, proceeding in turn to explain why the screamingly apparent contradiction of Christ is not after all contradictory (despite the appearances). But in the present context, per Pawl's (for-purposes-of-debate) assumption, the apparent contradiction is not a logical impossibility; and so some explanation is required as to why true contradictions should be treated as impossible in theology. And we don't get that from Biel or, as far as I know, from any of the other mainstream (or even side-stream) theologians to which Pawl's argument points.

The first horn of Pawl's principal objection is that even if logic doesn't rule out true contradictory theories, true theology's own extra-logical consequence relation rules them out. Pawl's argument from theological practice – qua practice of the relevant experts – fails to establish his first horn. The argument fails to show that true theology has a consequence relation that treats contradictions as explosive sentences.

4.3.5.2 From mixing domains?

The second horn of Pawl's dilemma is that would-be contradictions in theology find their way into scientific theories that are governed by contradiction-exploding consequence relations. Pawl's second horn rests on the claim, which I endorse, that at least some of our true scientific theories rule out the theoretical possibility of gluts; their consequence relations $\vdash_T$ validate explosion for contradictions: $!A \vdash_T B$. In particular, biology, I say in Beall 2019a, appears to be one such example; and Pawl relies on this example in the second argument for his principal claim.[29]

How does Pawl support his second horn? Pawl's strategy, if I understand it correctly, is to derive, from the contradictory case of Christ, a 'purely biological truth' which contradicts claims in (contradiction-exploding) biology; but since said derived truth is 'purely biological' it needs to be in the complete-as-possible true biology. But, then, true (and complete-as-possible) biology contains a contradiction; and true biology explodes in the face of contradictions. Hence, true biology is the trivial biology (viz., the theory containing all sentences in the language of biology). But we should reject the trivial biology and reject the root that led us to it – namely, Contradictory Christology.

What 'purely biological truth' is derivable from the contradictory case of Christ? Pawl gestures at many candidates but explicitly focuses on one: namely,

1. It is false that all humans have bodily parts.[30]

The argument for (1)? Here:

2. It's true that Christ is divine. [axiomatic in theology]

---

[29] One could use other sciences, except maybe mathematics; but biology is a good one.

[30] I change Pawl's example slightly to make plain that by 'has a body' Pawl means only 'has some bodily part'. (I also change to make the quantificational aspect of his example clear, and I drop the 'living adult human beings' to just 'humans', leaving any necessary tweaks – including potentially necessary reference to *actual* humans etc. – to be implicit. None of these changes affect his example or his overall strategy.)

   3. It's true that Christ is immaterial. [2; divinity entails immateriality]
   4. It's false that Christ has a bodily part. [3; immateriality entails so]
   5. It's true that Christ is human. [axiomatic in theology]
   1. It's false that all humans have bodily parts. [4, 5; logic (quantification)]

(1) is certainly a striking claim in the face of contemporary biological theory, but the argument for it – notwithstanding potential questions about divinity entailing immateriality – is solid. And this, Pawl argues, is the downfall of Contradictory Christology.

As Pawl's discussion makes clear, the argument towards (1) is constructed 'in the theology building' (so to speak). This isn't to say that in the theology building the true theories of other (non-theological) phenomena aren't invoked; they are – of course. For example, true theology contains at least some facts from true biology about humans, and at least some facts from true arithmetic, and at least some facts from true physics. These truths are developed and recorded in separate theories (viz., true biology, true arithmetic, true physics); but the truths from such theories are often lifted – as underived, ancillary truths – in theology. (And the same goes for biology lifting from physics, physics from analysis, etc.) All such inter-disciplinary lifting is common and uncontroversial. The showstopper that Pawl advances is that theology doesn't just contain – via lifting – truths from biology; theology itself is a source for biological truth! Theology itself, according to Pawl's argument, derives (let me say) 'purely biological truths' that couldn't be derived 'in the biology building' alone.

I think that Pawl's argument is very important and equally interesting but ultimately fails to establish its target. The reason, in short, is that (1) is 'purely biological' only if all of the entities over which it quantifies are 'purely biological', and in particular only if divine entities count as 'purely biological entities'. The problem, in the end, may be seen via a distinction. Distinguish 'normal biology' from 'abnormal biology' (and similarly for other theoretical domains), where the domain of the former is devoid of gods, and the domain of the latter includes the domain of the former but also contains some divine entities. With this distinction in hand the background assumption about true biological theory – which is central to Pawl's running argument – is to be rephrased: true normal biology is explosive with respect to contradictions, but true abnormal biology is no more explosive with respect to contradictions than true theology. In turn, Pawl's derivation of (1) is a derivation common to both true theology and true abnormal biology;

but the contradiction isn't explosive in abnormal biology, and so the case does not play the intended role against Contradictory Christology (and its alleged effect on true biology).

4.3.6 The role of logic in theology

In §2 and elsewhere it's claimed that the role of logic (-al consequence) in theology is its role in all truth-seeking disciplines: namely, to serve as the foundational or basement-level closure relation at the bottom of all true theories (specifically, at the bottom of the theories' closure relations). This claim, about logic and its role, is the chief target of a discussion by A. J. Cotnoir:

> I want to challenge the idea that the role of logic in theology is as Beall suggests. Theologians should, I argue, think of logical methods as a set of *tools* for constructing (closed) theories, and not as a universal *foundation* for all possible theories. (Cotnoir, 2019)

It appears that if Cotnoir's claim is correct then the claims about logical consequence in §2 are wrong.

Reply. The issue is largely terminological, as far as I can see.

Assume, as I claim in §2, that logical consequence is the consequence (closure) relation at the bottom of each true theory's own consequence relation; it's the one that governs the logical vocabulary, which is the vocabulary common to the languages of all of our true and complete-as-possible theories. In a picture, think of all true theories lined up in a row, each paired with their respective consequence relation (the closure relation under which the theories are closed or 'completed'):

$$\langle T_1, \vdash_{T_1} \rangle, \langle T_2, \vdash_{T_2} \rangle, \dots, \langle T_n, \vdash_{T_n} \rangle$$

Each such consequence relation $\vdash_{T_i}$ is a theory-specific entailment relation which governs the language of the given true theory T_i. The question is: where is *logic* in all this? Where, in other words, is *logical consequence* in this parade of theory-specific consequence relations? The answer that I've given – which, perhaps I should note, is entirely traditional and in no way non-standard or radical in the context of the question at hand – is that logical consequence (logic, for short) is in each and every such $\vdash_{T_i}$;[31] logic is at the bottom of each theory's consequence relation, governing the logical vocabulary (and only the logical vocabulary). Logic, in this way, is 'universal' and 'topic-neutral', involved in the consequence relation of every true (and complete-as-possible) theory. The sense in which logic is involved is so-called extensional: that if $X \therefore A$ is logically valid (i.e., if the sentences in X jointly entail sentence A according to logic) then $X \therefore A$ is T_i-valid too (i.e., then X entails A according to $\vdash_{T_i}$ too).

Now to Cotnoir's claim: 'theologians should think of logical methods as a set of tools for constructing closed theories, and not as a universal foundation for all possible theories' (Cotnoir, 2019). I agree with this as a statement about *logical methods*, and indeed as a statement about the vast multitude of consequence relations (qua closure relations) defined over the many languages of many theories. I have no disagreement whatsoever with Cotnoir's claim, so given. But the issue to which my discussion of logic's role is directed in §2 is not an issue concerning the role of *logical methods*; the issue concerns the role of 'universal closure' or basement-level consequence (entailment, closure) in all of our true theories.

There is a multitude of consequence relations on any given language – at least any given natural language. In the field of logic, any relation that remotely looks like a consequence relation – or that can be modeled in a way that remotely resembles a consequence relation – is called 'a logic'.[32] This terminology is good in many contexts but not so good in others. One context in which the usage is regrettable concerns debates over whether logic is subclassical (or non-classical in some other fashion), debates that are directly relevant to the topic of contradictory theology. Here, the debate is not whether there are logical methods that result in interesting and fruitful accounts of subclassical entailment relations. (Of course there are – many many times over.) Moreover, the debate is not whether such subclassical 'logics' can be used to do interesting modeling work in various theoretical pursuits. (Again, of course they can because they are so used – many many times over.) Accordingly, the debate over whether logic is subclassical is something else.

---

[31] Unless otherwise stated, it should be plain that when I'm talking about logic I'm talking about logical consequence – not the field of logic, not 'logical methods' (a bit more on which below), or etc.

[32] For a sense of the 5-fold field of contemporary logic see my Oxford Bibliographies article with John P. Burgess entitled 'Logic' (Beall and Burgess, 2017).

One might think that debates about whether logic is subclassical (versus classical) are about 'good reasoning' or rational acceptance–rejection behavior in our search for true theories. But this is not correct, at least for current debates over subclassical logic. Any account of the structure of rational acceptance–rejection behavior – any account of 'good reasoning' that is involved in our search for true theories – must reflect the sort of take-back (technically, non-monotonic) feature which is salient in the given structure. For example, our true theory of 'good reasoning' in our search for true theories may be such that all claims in set X jointly count as 'good reason' to accept the truth of A, but if you add some particular B to X the result of this union, namely, $X \cup \{B\}$, fails to count as a good reason for A; indeed, $X \cup \{B\}$ might well count as a good reason to reject A, and not merely fail to be good reason to accept A. The relation governing our rational pursuit of true theories is not itself a so-called monotonic one, and is thereby not an entailment or consequence relation at all. But current debates over whether logic is subclassical are debates over entailment relations – all of the leading candidates lack the sort of take-back, non-monotonic structure.

As I have said elsewhere (Beall, 2015, 2018), I accept what I take to be largely uncontroversial in contemporary philosophy of logic, namely, the distinction between an account of logic (qua consequence or entailment relation) and an account of 'good reasoning' or rational acceptance–rejection behavior. This distinction is not new or even recent but it was made very explicit in the work of Gilbert Harman (1999, 1986), work with which I'm largely in agreement (not about the details of the true account of logic but on the given distinctions). For present purposes, it is worth being even more explicit that the debate over whether logic is subclassical is not a debate over the very important but equally messy phenomenon of rational acceptance–rejection behavior. Of course, like just about any sufficiently fundamental issues, the true account of one of the given phenomena (e.g., logic) bears in many ways on the true account of the other (e.g., rational acceptance–rejection behavior); but such is our messy epistemic situation, no matter the phenomena of concern.

Debates about whether logic is subclassical (versus classical) are important and pressing debates. I've briefly indicated (above) what those debates are not about. The question remains: what, then, is being debated when we debate whether logic is subclassical? The answer to which I've pointed is as above: the debate is over which candidate consequence relation (viz., some given subclassical relation or the mainstream so-called classical candidate) plays the role of 'universal closure' or 'universal consequence' in all of our true theories – which of the candidates is the one on top of which our many theory-specific consequence relations are built? If the answer is the mainstream (i.e., classical) candidate, then any contradictory theory (a fortiori, any contradictory theology) is the trivial one, since each theory's consequence relation obeys logic (since each theory has logic at the foundation of its own closure relation), and the mainstream candidate has it that any arbitrary contradiction logically entails any arbitrary sentence in the language of the theory.[33] On the other hand, if, as I hold, the answer is a suitable subclassical candidate where arbitrary !A fails to entail arbitrary B then not all contradictory theories need be trivial theories.

Cotnoir's principal challenge to the foregoing (and, again, very standard, traditional) characterization of the role of logic (-al consequence) in all true theories is in fact not a challenge to the given characterization. There might be a challenge to my characterization were Cotnoir to argue that the role of universal closure on all true theories is played by not one consequence relation but rather many, whatever that might come to. I am not sure what such a position would involve unless it were some crude sort of relativism – some crude sort of anything-goes-ism – about the entailments of our true and complete-as-possible theories; however, Cotnoir explicitly rejects such a relativism (Cotnoir, 2019, §4.2).

By way of summary let me be crystal clear in my reply to Cotnoir's would-be challenge: Cotnoir's given challenge is a challenge that doesn't apply to my position; it's a challenge, if I understand it correctly, to the view that logical methods are not to be seen as useful theoretical tools. I stand with Cotnoir in firmly – firmly, firmly, firmly – holding that the techniques, methods, and tools of logic (qua field of study) are extraordinarily useful modeling ingredients applicable to all disciplines, from theology to biology and everywhere in between. While it's unlikely that one particular tool or method or technique will be of equal value in its modeling work across all disciplines, it is equally unlikely that no such tool or method or technique will be of any value. On this Cotnoir and I – and, I strongly suspect, just about all researchers in and around logic (qua field) – agree. This is an important point for analytic theology (and any other truth-seeking discipline); but it does not

---

[33] As a reminder on terminology: the *trivial theory in a language L* is the theory containing all sentences of L. A *contradiction in L* is any sentence in L of the form $\dagger A \wedge \neg A$ or, logically equivalently, $A \wedge \neg A$ (sometimes abbreviated !A) where $\dagger$ is logic's (logically redundant) truth connective (viz., 'it is true that . . . ') and $\neg$ is logic's falsity connective (viz., 'it is false that . . . ', also called *logical negation*).

in any way challenge my account of the role of logic (-al consequence) in true theories – including the true theology.

4.4 Metaphysical issues

4.4.1 On the charge of 'shifting the focus off Christ'

In §3.4 it is claimed that pointing to Christ's 'parts' (broadly construed) en route to a consistent account carries the defect of shifting the focus off of Christ, and onto Christ's 'parts' (broadly construed). §3.4 likewise claims that, on such accounts, Christ ultimately bears the divine and human properties 'only by charity', and that this is objectionable. But this isn't any different from the common 'four-dimensionalist' view of our sitting, standing, and so forth. On those views, we are four-dimensional spacetime 'worms' made up, at least in significant part, by 'time slices' of our ourselves. Some person exemplified the property of *sitting* this morning in virtue of her given temporal part's sitting at just that time, and she exemplified the property of *not sitting* this evening in virtue of another of her temporal part's standing – or at any rate, not sitting – this evening. And there's nothing objectionable about this familiar account around the otherwise contradictory exemplification of *sitting and not sitting*.[34]

Reply. There are at least three replies, each of which, on my view, sufficiently rebuts the running objection (or the running defense of shifting-subjects routes towards consistentizing Christ).

First, as far as I can see, the would-be defense is a concession that Christ doesn't really have – or at least only-by-charity has – the core divine and human properties. After all, this is the case with the four-dimensionalist position: *you* don't in fact exemplify *sitting*; rather, various other things *that are not you* exemplify *sitting.* You by-charity exemplify sitting, which only requires having a suitably related part that in fact sits. 'Translating', then, Christ doesn't exemplify the divine or human properties; Christ only by-charity does, piggybacking on the work of other entities not one of which is Christ. And that's what I said: the central properties of Christ are now not really Christ's but, according to such shifting-subjects views, properties of

---

[34] Mike Rea put this point to me in conversation, as did Tim Pawl in comments on a previous draft. This shifting-subject objection arises again in §5.

things not one of which is Christ. Christ, as I said, has the divine and human properties only by charity. And this, as per the shifting-focus objection, is at best unmotivated, at least when the contradictory option keeps the focus squarely on Christ as the bearer (and not by-charity bearer) of the key divine and human properties.

Second, the cases behind the defense are critically different. In the four-dimensionalist case, you *are the wrong sort of thing* to sit, stand and so forth; you're just the spacetime worm that's simply the wrong kind of thing to satisfy 'sits', 'stands' and so forth, and not the wrong kind of thing at this time or that time but the wrong kind of thing – full stop. For the analogy to be strong, Christ needs to be the wrong kind of thing to bear the divine and human properties – and not just the wrong kind of thing at this time or that time but the wrong kind of thing – full stop. And this strikes me not only as seriously questionable; it's also without motivation, except for the apparent contradiction that would otherwise result from Christ's bearing the target divine and human properties.

Third, the only reason the shifting-subject views shift the subject is the apparent contradiction of Christ. Unlike the case of 'sitting' and 'standing' over time, wherein there's no claim of any particular time that you sit and don't sit, the case of Christ is very much different: he is said to be divine (and all that that entails) and human (and all that that entails) *at one and the same time*, for many, many, many such times. Not so for some t and your sitting and not sitting. In the case of Christ, the apparent contradiction is affirmed of many (many) particular times: Christ is mutable and immutable at t. Such is the claim. Such is the apparent contradiction. Were there not many times of which Christ is said to be both divine and human (and all that being so entails) then resisting the contradiction at the cost of some by-charity exemplification might be well motivated. But there are many such times. And so shifting the focus to other entities strikes me as accordingly unmotivated, at least when the contradictory account is clearly viable.

4.4.2 Observable contradictions?

Contradictory Christology seems to be committed to contradictory beings in the observable world. The idea of 'observable gluts' requires elaboration. As Pawl (2019*a*) observes:

According to Contradictory Christology, Christ is not mutable, in the ordinary sense of that term. Christ cannot, and did not, change. Now, one question here is, 'what did that look like, in real life?' Someone put a nail next to the flesh of his blessed hand, then struck the nail with a hammer. Did the nail pierce the skin? Yes, it did. But did it also not pierce the skin, owing to the fact that to be pierced is to change, and Christ did not change? Given that Contradictory Christology is an attempt at a general answer to the Fundamental Problem, what holds for mutability should hold for materiality, and for all the other instances of difficult predicates for Christology: passible, contingent, temporal, etc. What does it look like for something not material – not material in the sense of being the contradictory of material; not material in the same sense that the number 2 or the form of Courage is not material – to be struck? It seems to me that the contradictions proliferate at an astounding rate. He bled and he didn't; he walked on water and he didn't; he had a body and he didn't. Everything he did in life that required being incarnate is also something that he did not do, owing to the fact that he was not material, passable, mutable, and temporal. As [an] autobiographical note, I have a hard time picturing in my mind what it would look like to be around Jesus.   (Pawl, 2019a)

The issue/question is then just this: what do you say about observable gluts?

Reply. Before turning directly to the main issue of observable gluts, it is worth flagging that the 'astounding' spread of would-be contradictions to which Pawl points may not be nearly as widespread or astounding as portrayed. One reason, similar to the issues discussed in §4.3.1 above, is that the entailments on which Pawl's portrait depends may not contrapose in ways that underwrite the would-be spread of gluts. (Example: Pawl cites the entailment from 'pierced' to 'changes', and then invokes 'unchanging' to derive 'not pierced' – a valid derivation only if the given entailment relation contraposes, which is doubtful.) For that reason, I do not grant the proliferation of gluts that Pawl's comments presuppose, nor grant any of the particular cases that Pawl lists. I remain without a firm answer on exactly what features of the contradictory Christ Jesus are observable features.

There is a great deal more to be said about observable contradictions than can be said here. I address two issues: one, the dialectical role that the issue of observable contradictions might be taken to play; the other is simply the direction of my current thoughts on the issue of any would-be observable contradictions of Christ. I take each in turn.[35]

4.4.2.1 Note on dialectical role

An important dialectical point to keep in mind: one might try to argue from the absence of anticipated observable consequences of $A \wedge \neg A$ (as elsewhere, $!A$) to a rejection of $!A$. The thinking, for example, might be this: we know what it looks like when A is true; we know what it looks like when A is false; and so we know what it looks like when $!A$ is true, since $!A$ is true just if A is true and A is false. But for the alleged christological $!A$ we see only the observable consequences of A, or only the observable consequences of $\neg A$; and hence we should reject that $!A$ is true since its observable consequences are absent.

The would-be argument is not a good one. The success of such an argument rests squarely on facts concerning the observable consequences of $!A$. One might insist that the observable consequences of a conjunction just are the observable consequences of its conjuncts. But even if that's generally true, the claim is at least doubtful when it comes to contradictions, which, after all, tend to have (what else to say) 'contradictory consequences' – for example, that the cat is on the mat, that it's false that the cat is on the mat, and so on. If there were very strong reasons to think that the observable consequences of gluts just are the observable consequences of both conjuncts then – provided that Christ's contradictory properties have observable effects – we'd have a swift argument against Contradictory Christology in the absence of the required observable effects. But pending discovery of such very strong reasons for thinking that the observable consequences of gluts just are the observable consequences of both conjuncts, I think that the point remains doubtful.

From my perspective, there is very strong reason to think that Christ is contradictory (e.g., among other potential ones, the longstanding fundamental-problem arguments); but there's also strong reason to think that those who observed the crucifixion did not observe anything out of the ordinary (no would-be flittering between blood and absence of blood, or a nail hole and the absence of a nail hole, or any other flickering-buffering

---

[35] My reply here is intended to clarify what I now think is an ill-worded response found in Beall *et al.* 2019. I am grateful to Tim Pawl, Tom McCall, Meghan Page, and Mitchell Mallary for forcing me to be clearer in my response on the issue of any would-be observable contradictions of Christ. My response here remains only partial.

magic); they saw the blood, oozing from the nail holes, and so on – full stop. But rather than infer – in light of the ordinary observable consequences and lack of extraordinary 'flickering' or whathaveyou – that therefore there's no contradiction we should instead infer the more immediate fact: namely, that our expectations about the would-be observable consequence were unfounded. As such, it is not – nor has it ever been – that we look to its observable consequences to conclude that a phenomenon is contradictory; we rather look to a broader set of data, including, in the case at hand, revelation, the creeds, councils, reflection, and more.

While there is a very interesting and important issue concerning the observable consequences of Christ's contradictory being, the dialectical role that the issue plays is not a simple one from the absence of extraordinary observable consequences to the absence of the given contradiction.

* Parenthetical remark. Lest some readers are wondering, the epistemology of all this is not intended to be different from the epistemology of other truths. The truth about epistemology of just about anything is messy and hard; I see no reason to think that epistemology is wildly different in the case of a contradictory theology from the case of non-contradictory theology, except for underlying entailment relations under which the two theories are respectively closed. The topic of a systematic, logic-bound contradictory theology has been largely unexplored, and so surprises are likely; however, at least as yet, I see no reason to think that the epistemology of Contradictory Christology requires breaking genuinely new epistemological ground. *End remark.*

4.4.2.2 Initial thoughts on Christ's would-be observable contradictions

Setting aside the dialectical issues, the driving question remains: what, if any, are the observable consequences of Christ's contradictory truths? I do not, as yet, have a full answer, but the direction of my answer is strongly apparent in the discussion above (see §4.4.2.1).

That Christ is a contradictory being is not itself observable in the way in which Christ's blood is observable. From the fact that Christ Jesus was observed in ordinary empirical ways, it follows that some properties of Christ have observable consequences (i.e., that Christ's having *those* properties has observable consequences). But that any two of Christ's contradictory properties are jointly observable requires argument. The argument cannot proceed on the assumption that such and such observable consequences are involved in the case of all non-contradictory beings. That might be so, but the argument needs to apply to contradictory beings. And, to my knowledge, we simply don't have anything to go on here except for the extraordinary case of Christ, all of whose observable effects (in the usual, simple, flat-footed sense of 'observable effects') appear to be truly – and fully – describable without contradiction.

What you see (in general, empirically observe) in the contradictory Christ are the seeable features of the contradiction. Some of the observable features are clear: hanging on the cross, having a pierced side that was touchable after his resurrection, bleeding, and other known features. None of those, themselves or jointly, are contradictory. But the contradictory properties, entailed by Christ's divinity, are not clearly seeable or, generally, observable in the same way.

My conjecture is that the contradictory Christ – a walking, talking contradictory being – has no observable contradictory properties (in the usual sense of 'observable properties'). Indeed, of Christ's contradictory pairs of properties, it may well be that few of his divine properties have observable effects in the relevant sense. But this is neither surprising nor problematic. The truth of Christ's changing – being pierced, undergoing excruciating suffering, being striped with blood – is observable; it was observed by witnesses. And what was observed appeared as horrible as we would normally expect – not some flickering magical image that in any way appeared less than the stench of the crucifixion. What was observed smelled as horrible as we would normally take it to smell. There was nothing that lightens the severity of the truth of Christ's given changes. Nothing. On the other hand, the immutability of Christ – the falsity of Christ's mutability – is not something that we see, smell or touch in the same flat-footed sense of 'see', 'smell', and so on. But, again, there's nothing magical here: Christ is mutable and immutable; Christ changes but it's false that Christ changes. How this contradiction *looks* turns on the observable effects of Christ's having the given properties. What was seen, on gruesome display, was the truth of Christ's changing, the truth of Christ's severe suffering; what was not seen (in the same sense of 'see') were any observable effects of Christ's divine contradictory properties – his immutability, for example. But the truth of Christ's mutability neither undermines nor diminishes the falsity of Christ's mutability; we simply see only the seeable – more generally, observable – effects of whichever properties, in that combination, have observable consequences. And Christ's immutability (for example) is not among the seeable properties in his given pool of contradictory properties, at least for all that was empirically witnessed.

4.4.3 Metaphysical neutrality (I)

It is claimed in §3 that a virtue of Contradictory Christology over other accounts is metaphysical neutrality. But Contradictory Christology is hardly metaphysically neutral; it requires the truth of contradictions, beings who are contradictory! This is a serious metaphysical commitment, and hardly a metaphysically neutral feature of the theory.[36]

Reply. Every true theory is committed to whatever is entailed by the theory – entailed by the given truths. Contradictory Christology is no different. The only would-be difference is that true consistent theories (e.g., many of our true theories in science, mathematics, or whathaveyou) have non-contradictory consequences; any true contradictory theory – including any true contradictory christology – has contradictory consequences. But there's no difference in 'metaphysical commitment' in any of this. The only difference is that on the contradictory account there are aspects – rare and exceedingly special aspects – of reality that are truly described by falsehoods (though not by falsehoods that aren't also truths). But there's nothing in this that demands a stake in any particular metaphysical theory in the way that other theories – particularly 'quest'-driven christological theories – have a stake in particular metaphysical theories. Such accounts pin the truth (because the alleged consistency) of Christ on the truth of one or another metaphysical theory. Contradictory Christology does no such thing, at least as far as I can see.

One might push the current objection by pointing to the demand for 'negative facts' in the world, and that such 'facts' are clearly metaphysically rich entities to which no genuinely metaphysically neutral theory is committed. But even on this pushing-further point, the objection overstates the case.

There are two senses of 'facts' that are relevant: one is the redundant one, sharing the so-called transparency of so-called transparent truth

---

[36] A version of this objection was raised by A. J. Cotnoir in his presented comments on a paper of mine delivered at the *Logos* Institute at the University of St. Andrews (though Cotnoir should not in any way be taken to endorse the objection as I've given it).

(Beall, 2019*b*); the other is a sort of 'correspondence' or 'truth-making' and 'falsity-making' sense. Take each in turn.

On the transparent sense of 'fact', there's nothing more nor less, entailment-wise, to the claims

- That grass is green is a fact
- That pigs don't fly is a fact

than, respectively,

- Grass is green.
- Pigs don't fly.

If one persists in asking 'what is this fact that grass is green?' or 'what is this fact that pigs don't fly?', my response, relying on the transparent notion of 'fact', is as before: it's that grass is green; it's that pigs don't fly. If one wants further consequences of these facts, one can explore the entailments of grass' being green (a subject of various sciences, presumably) or the entailments of pigs not flying (a subject of various sciences, including physics and biology). But to press more is to press for something that requires argument – argument for why we should expect there to be more than this.

On the 'correspondence' (say, truth-making, falsity-making) sense of 'fact', one is supposed to be talking about metaphysical bits and bobs in the world that 'make true' and 'make false' our various truths and falsehoods. And this is certainly, at least traditionally, a field of philosophy (and, in some ways, systematic theology) thick in lots of metaphysical theory. But on this sense of 'facts', the prior question remains: why do we need such entities in our account of the true theory of reality? (Frankly, the answer remains very unclear to me.) Pending a good answer, it's not obvious that 'negative facts' – the entities posited as falsity-making bits of the world – are necessary for contradictory truths, since it's not obvious that any such 'correspondence entities' (so to speak) are required.

Finally, and still on the 'correspondence' sense of 'fact', suppose that there's good reason to find an account of entities in the world that make our claims true (including making negations true, that is, making our claims false). Well, if this is required of the true theory of reality then it's required; and we need to find truth- and falsity-makers in the world for our true claims (ergo, our true negative claims). I see no reason to think that Contradictory Christology is saddled with any peculiar problem here unless non-contradictory (i.e., consistent) theories contain no negations in them at all – a very unlikely prospect.

I conclude, then, that the running objection should be rejected: Contradictory Christology is metaphysically neutral in significant ways, especially when compared with 'metaphysical' routes on the quest to consistentize Christ.[37]

4.4.4 Metaphysical neutrality (II)

It is claimed in §3.3 that a virtue of Contradictory Christology over other accounts is metaphysical neutrality.[38] The claim, in particular, is this:

> [A] very strong methodological principle [is] that, in the absence of an officially stamped revealed metaphysics, a metaphysically neutral solution to the fundamental 'problem' of christology – to the apparent contradiction of Christ – is better than one whose viability depends on the would-be truth of a specific metaphysical theory.

We can parody this with 'Logical neutrality' rather than 'Metaphysical neutrality' just so:

> [A] very strong methodological principle [is] that, in the absence of an officially stamped revealed logic, a logically neutral solution to the fundamental 'problem' of christology – to the apparent contradiction of Christ – is better than one whose viability depends on the would-be truth of a specific logical theory.

But, now, in such a case your theory – demanding a subclassical account of logic – is worse than a logically neutral one.

Reply. There are at least two replies. First, no true theory is logically neutral, since all true theories are closed under logic. In this way, logic is special in a way that metaphysics isn't, and in just this respect the given parity-of-

---

[37] While not in response to the running objection on metaphysical neutrality, but lest there be doubt on the matter, I note that there are very simple accounts of 'falsity-making' entities sufficient for the 'correspondence' project (Beall, 2000).

[38] A version of this objection was raised by Laura Frances Callahan during a Center for Philosophy of Religion workshop at Notre Dame.

reasoning objection fails. Second, even setting aside the first reply (which, in fact, should not be set aside), the objection ultimately undermines the mainstream account of logic in favor of something approaching the so-called nil account of logic (viz., where there are no logically valid forms, and every entailment that turns on logical vocabulary is validated only by theory-specific consequence relations).[39] The objection, in this case, motivates a subclassical account of logical consequence that is perfectly compatible with a true contradictory christology.

4.4.5   Christ as unique source of contradictions?

In previous chapters it is claimed that Christ is the unique contradictory being, but that's untrue. Take anyone who prays to Christ, and therefore is related by prayer to a contradictory being. Then it's true that the praying subject prays to one who is omniscient (since it's true that Christ is omniscient), but it's also false that the praying subject prays to one who is omniscient (since it's false that Christ is omniscient).[40] Hence, all who pray to Christ – or, indeed, are related to Christ in many other ways – are themselves contradictory beings, since there are claims that are true and false of them. But, then, Christ is hardly the unique contradictory being – a consequence that belies the would-be conservativeness of Contradictory Christology with respect to contradictory beings.

Reply. My principal claim is not that Christ is the unique contradictory being; the claim is that Christ – the GodMan – is the source of contradictory beings.[41] So, even if all Christians wind up as derivatively contradictory beings – deriving their contradictory-being status from their various relations to Christ – the principal claim remains true (and, I note, duly conservative with respect to the source of contradictory beings).

---

[39] For technical reasons, the would-be nil 'logic' doesn't count as a candidate for logic qua universal closure relation (defined over standard vocabulary) on all true theories, since it won't be reflexive (assuming, as I do, that true theories have at least one true claim in them, and that all claims in a true theory are true – even if some may also be false), but for purposes of the objection I set this aside. For discussion in the direction of nil-logic-related issues see the work of Cotnoir (2018*a*), French (2016), and Russell (2018).

[40] A version of this objection was given by Thomas Hofweber during discussion of my work at the *Logos* Institute in St. Andrews.

[41] I do not count the comparatively uninteresting linguistic-level gluts – the spandrels of 'true' or the like (Beall, 2009) – among contradictory beings. If it adds clarity, the claim is that Christ is the source of 'metaphysical contradiction' versus 'linguistic contradiction' in the world, though the distinction is ultimately a hard one to spell out. (I flag this only to set it aside.)

But there's also more to say. The objection rests on an incorrect step. The objection seems to rely on a 'commutativity' principle that goes from the falsity of a true contradiction to the falsity of standing in a binary relation to the given contradictory being. In the particular case at hand, we have the following truths:

i. It's true that Christ is omniscient.
ii. It's false that Christ is omniscient.
iii. Christians pray to Christ.
iv. Christians pray to a being (viz., Christ) who is omniscient.

But how do we get from the foregoing truths to the target 'spread' objection? The objection requires the truth of

* It's false that Christians pray to a being (viz., Christ) who is omniscient.

But where does (*) come from? If the falsity operator (i.e., logical negation) commuted with the prayer relation then (*) follows, with minimal fiddling (e.g., so-called existential generalization on 'Christ'), from (ii). But I see no reason to think that the prayer relation in particular or, more importantly, any relevant binary relation commutes with logical negation in the given way. Pending reason to think as much, I conclude that the objection fails to show even that Christians (or any other objects) are derivatively contradictory beings; true theories – such as the true christology – have consequence relations that invalidate the given commutation behavior.

4.5 Ecumenical issues

4.5.1 How does this serve apologetics?

How is Contradictory Christology apologetically helpful?[42] Suppose some atheist accepts the following two claims:

A0. Subclassical logic is correct.
A1. There are gluts (i.e., some contradictions are true).

---

[42] This objection/question was raised by Jeremy Sakovich in written correspondence.

It does not follow from either (or both) of these, if assumed to be true, that the person who is committed to them is also thereby committed to the view that Contradictory Christology is true. There is still required further argument to demonstrate at least two more claims:

i. The claims of christology are contradictions.
ii. Said contradictions in (i) are gluts.

Now, it's easy enough to think that an atheist will find themselves committed to (i), but why should any such atheist lend credence to (ii)? Contradictory Christology only pushes the debate with atheists and non-Christians to a different point: namely, defining and articulating the conditions under which a contradiction is true (likewise, false), how we should become aware of such conditions, and so on. But, then, instead of demonstrating that christology is consistent and the contradictions contained within are only apparent, if Contradictory Christology is true, the apologist must now shoulder the burden of demonstrating to the unbeliever that the contradiction of Christ is true. This will prove difficult precisely because the contradictions of christology strike non-Christians as clearly false – or worse, as nonsense. Indeed, the contradictions of christology serve as reasons in arguments for rejecting the christian account of reality.

Reply. Apologists for christian theology defend the truth of the christian theory of reality. That's what they *should* be doing. Apologetics should not be thought of as a game of winning a debate. Moreover, on my view, it's not for the apologist to convince an atheist or even agnostic or even a non-christian theist of the truth of the given theory. The truth is what it is, and the truth can speak for itself – often in mysterious ways, as christian tradition long affirms. The task of apologetics, when properly done, is simply to defend the theory against precise objections; it's not to persuade. (If it were, apologists should first set their principal target on the christian church itself – the universal but wildly diverse church – and specifically on its divisions. Here at least there is unity in a commitment to finding the true christian theology, but as history and ongoing practice shows, strong divisions remain as a reflection of apparent failure to persuade. But, again, the role of apologetics, as I see it, is not persuasion; it's defense, and defense only in the face of clear – versus vaguely gestured – objection.)

Is there any way in which the truth of A0 and A1 serve apologetics? Well, adjusting A1 to A2, namely,

A2. The true theory of Christ is contradictory (i.e., glutty).

'defends' against the fundamental 'problem' of christology – which is at the heart of the christian theory of reality. How so? Well, it's hardly an objection to repeat the theory's main thesis.

Who 'wins' the debate? As above, I've truly no interest whatsoever in that question – absolutely none. If an atheist (or agnostic or non-christian theist) charges that the christian theory (per Chalcedon at least) is contradictory, I say: correct. If the would-be objector then points out that the theory cannot thereby be rationally endorsed, I ask for an explanation. For all I've seen, there's still no good explanation as to why the would-be objector's given claim is correct.

Similarly, if the atheist (or agnostic or non-christian theist) charges that christian theory is flat-out nonsense, I respond: how so? And I'd sincerely want the answer. Pending a precise answer that shows – contrary to all appearances – the alleged nonsense, there's little more that can or need be said. An apologist of the christian theory (indeed, if I'm right, the true contradictory theory) should not be engaged in trying to persuade the would-be objector that the theory is true (and, therefore, full of sense, so to speak); she should focus on clearly articulated objections that demand a defense of the truth. Because of the dogmatic attitudes against gluts, based largely or wholly on a weak account of logic (-al consequence) itself, some sincere would-be objectors might think that contradictions – the logical conjunction of a sentence and its logical negation – are meaningless (i.e., nonsense). This is an important concern to answer and indeed refute. (One first step in refutation: if meaningless, then they cannot stand on either side of logical entailment; but even by the mainstream account of logical entailment, an arbitrary contradiction $!A$ entails all sentences, and is both by itself and as part – that is, subsentence – entailed by a variety of sentences. Some of the other steps are in various parts of this book.)

4.5.2   Historically suspect

The proposal is historically suspect. According to Gregory Dunn, Leo the Great maintained that 'Jesus could be both impassible and passible at the same time *without there being any contradiction*' [emphasis mine] Dunn (2001).[43] Hence, inasmuch as Dunn's interpretation of Leo is correct, and

---

[43] This quotation is used by Pawl (2016) for different dialectical purposes, but the passage nicely frames the current objection. I discuss an importantly related objection, based on Pawl's work, below.

in turn Leo's texts were ratified as part of at least any orthodox Catholic christology, the proposed contradictory christology is historically suspect.

Reply. Distinguish two senses of 'contradiction', one being a sentence which is the logical conjunction of a sentence and its logical negation, and the other being an 'explosive sentence', a sentence that, according to a theory's consequence or entailment relation, entails every sentence (of the language of the theory). The first sense is the one involved in the proposed Contradictory Christology. I agree with Dunn and many others that the true christology has no true explosive sentences – that is, no claims that are both true according to the christology and also entail all sentences according to the christology's consequence relation. So, there is nothing in Contradictory Christology, as I've advanced it, that conflicts with the (Dunn reading of) the Leo claims.

Also, just to be perfectly clear, Contradictory Christology, as I'm advancing it, is – for all that I can see – compatible with orthodox Catholic christology (and theology, generally), at least as a candidate true theory of Christ; however, the account is not advanced within the narrowly defined 'Conciliar Christology' (and its full methodological commitments) as defined and developed by Pawl (2016, 2019b). By my lights, Pawl's Conciliar Christology is one of many candidate theories for the true christology, to be measured and assessed along with the others.

4.5.3 Hermeneutically suspect

The proposal is hermeneutically suspect by being uncharitable in reading conciliar texts, specifically in the contradictory reading of Chalcedon (451). Pawl (2014), focused only on his Conciliar Christology (with which, as a candidate theory, my proposal is intended to be compatible), implicitly argues that it's *uncharitable* to charge the Chalcedon thinkers with advancing a contradictory christology:

> Had they really believed these five pairs of predicates to be incompatible, they would not have affirmed that Christ is both visible and invisible, incomprehensible and comprehensible, unlimited and limited, impassible and passible, and inexpressible and expressible. It is a rare feat to be able to contradict oneself so forcefully in a single sentence. Any one of these five conjunctive pairs would be enough to entail a contradiction, and the fathers do it five times over!   (Pawl, 2014, p. 64)

The point is that it's at best uncharitable to interpret the conciliar fathers as advancing anything close to a genuinely contradictory christology.

Reply. Let me be explicit: the conciliar fathers may've erroneously thought that logic rules out a contradictory being, and hence rules out Christ's being a contradictory being. If they did, and if Catholics – or at least Conciliar Christians along the practice of Pawl's definition of 'Conciliar Christology' (Pawl, 2016) – are required to be in step with all theories held by conciliar fathers (including, therefore, their theory of logical consequence) then, to my deep disappointment, Contradictory Christology, as I've advanced it, is simply unavailable to Catholics so understood. But I find it very difficult to believe that Catholicism demands such in-step practice beyond core claims of Christ and God more generally. And if that's correct, I stand by the claim that a contradictory account of Christ is not only compatible with conciliar claims about Christ; it's the best reading.

One problem with Pawl's (charity-driven) hermeneutical argument comes with an uncharitable reading of the conciliar fathers. Either the Chalcedon 451 writers shirked the opportunity to flag their (as-yet-unresolved) alternative usage of the key predicates (e.g., 'passible' and 'impassible', etc.) or they used the predicates in their standard ways with their standard but glaringly contradictory consequences. Since, as Pawl (2019*a*) rightly points out, said writers seem to (mistakenly) think that contradictions are logically impossible, it's reasonable to interpret them as Pawl suggests: namely, as meaning something very different from the standard meanings, some very obviously non-contradictory usage of the target terms. But therein lies the rub. Charity demands that we take said thinkers to be aware of the apparent contradiction in what Chalcedon 451 ultimately affirms. One immediate question: why not simply and quickly put this appearance aside by flagging the non-standard or otherwise alternative usage that is supposed to be perfectly free of a contradictory reading?[44] One answer might be the conjecture that the clearly contradiction-free usage was so dominant at Chalcedon 451 that it was the default usage. Maybe, but such a substantial empirical claim demands equally substantial empirical evidence, and the history, to my knowledge, is at best unclear (at this time of writing, viz., 2019). (How on earth was such a

---

[44] The work of Cross (2019) shows that at least some much later thinkers, such as Gabriel Biel (15c), either constructed, perhaps in response to the apparent contradiction, or were otherwise familiar with non-standard satisfaction conditions for target terms (e.g., 'mutable' and 'immutable', etc.), satisfaction conditions that are *obviously* non-contradictory.

clearly critical usage lost or otherwise left to become non-standard?) Pending further evidence, I suggest that an alternative explanation is at hand. In particular, the more charitable reading of the Chalcedon writers (at least with respect to the key christological account) is that they saw no other way to account for the full reality of Christ except by using contradictory language. On this reading, the writers, being on the quest to consistentize Christ, erroneously reject the logical possibility of Christ's being a contradictory being; however, the reality of Christ's divinity and the reality of Christ's humanity and the reality of Christ's being exactly one person combined to jointly demand the contradictory language – *on pain of leaving out an important aspect of the reality of Christ's being.* The Chalcedon writers, along with many of those on the dominant and ongoing quest to consistentize Christ, rejected that contradictions could (logically) be true; however, the radical, scandalous reality of Christ demanded the resulting language, apparent contradiction and all. This, I think, is a more charitable reading of the situation than one according to which the default and widely dominant usage of target thinkers involved what, today, we consider to be non-standard satisfaction conditions for target terms.[45] In short, the writers wished that they had non-contradictory language to describe the full and apparently contradictory reality of Christ; they so wished because they equally firmly believed that contradictory beings are logically impossible. Still, to affirm anything less than the apparent contradiction (e.g., passible and impassible, mutable and immutable, etc.) is to leave something out of the true description, to at best misleadingly give a partial account. Instead, they wrote what the full reality of Christ demands: fully divine and fully human and just one person. And in the end, they saw a mystery in how this apparent contradiction could be true, but anything less would be misleadingly partial.[46]

---

[45] A terminological (and non-dialectical) aside: I should flag that Pawl, in his work (2016, 2019*b*), calls the target conditions 'truth conditions', but this is a very non-standard (and, as far as I can see, unmotivated) deviation from standard usage. (It's also unnecessary for his program.) Sentences have truth and falsity conditions, since sentences (not predicates) are true or false. *Predicates* are never true or false; they're *true of* or *false of* objects. (And when they're true of an object, then using that predicate together with a singular term for said object delivers a true sentence. Mutatis Mutandis for predicates that are false of an object, and false sentences.) The standard term in philosophy for 'true of' conditions is 'satisfaction conditions'. As far as I can see, there's no theological reason to change the standard philosophical terminology in this context.

[46] I note that the take of Sarah Coakley (2002) on Chalcedon 451 and other conciliar work sits well with this reading, at least inasmuch as her position is compatible with the contradictory truth of Christ.

To be clear, I am not taking a stand on the correct historical interpretation of the conciliar writers or their intentions or their mental states generally. My claim, by way of reply to the given objection, is that there's a more – or, perhaps, at least equally – charitable reading of the Chalcedon writers than the non-contradictory one advanced in the objection.[47]

4.5.4 Other theological contradictions

It looks like Contradictory Christology naturally generalizes to other parts of theology. In particular, doesn't the general proposal require that every apparent contradiction in theology be treated as contradictory – including, perhaps especially, the very familiar 'logical' puzzles involving God's omniscience, omnipotence (a too-heavy stone) and the like?

Reply. No. While logic leaves open such possibilities – and theologians should be aware of such logical possibilities – the contradiction needs to be motivated too. While the familiar 'logical' problems (Nagasawa, 2008, 2017) of the traditional 'omnigod' are candidates for a contradictory proposal (Cotnoir, 2018*b*), the contradiction involved is not as clear as the screamingly apparent contradiction of Christ's role and two natures. I do not rule out a contradictory resolution of other theological problems but, pending debate, my proposal is restricted to the fundamental problem of christology: namely, that Christ is the source of all (non-linguistic) contradictions in the world. I take up the question of a broader glut-theoretic (contradictory) theology in §6, where some directions towards the trinity result in theological gluts – namely, of God – arising not just from Christ but from differences among the divine persons.[48]

---

[47] Let me be very clear here: I am at best a first-rung novice on the history of the councils; so the foregoing is not in any way put forth as an attempt at historical record, a record that undoubtedly involves a great many truths about the political-cum-economic climate whirling around the given councils. That said, to explain away the clearly apparent contradictions as little more than disappointing political pandering strikes me as a very serious step backwards, a step that, pending the discovery of very good reason to make, I set aside entirely.

[48] As said elsewhere, I do not provide an official account of the trinity in this book. That is for a subsequent book devoted entirely to the trinity. §6 aims simply to sketch salient issues on that topic. For a sample gap-theoretic approach to standard 'logical' omni-property problems, see Beall and Cotnoir 2017.

4.5.5 Just highfalutin theory

This is all just highfalutin theory; it has nothing to do with the real work of christology or theology in general.

Reply. That's just wrong. Theologians are theoreticians who, if aiming to get at the true theory of God, seek to record not only the fundamental truths but also all *consequences* of those truths. And this requires that theologians construct an appropriate consequence (closure) relation for theology. And to do this the systematic theologian must take a stance on the fundamental closure relation: namely, logic itself. To think that it's obvious that logic is as per the standard account of logic (viz., so-called classical) is to think in error. Even defenders of the standard account of logic reject that it's obvious that logic is per the standard account.

Moreover, there is a genuine practical upside to Contradictory Christology. The role of Christ demands an entity who is not unlimited, one who can truly understand and experience our limited and imperfect ignorance of what it would be like to escape limitations (something we can only imperfectly imagine); but the role of Christ equally demands an entity who is devoid of limitations – the perfect and limitless God worthy of worship by all. The fundamental 'problem' of christology is that this role is contradictory; it demands realization at the price of a contradictory being. But Christians may rest assured that Christ is that contradiction: truly perfect; truly imperfect – all in the standard senses of those terms. Hiding the full force of Christ's contradictory being by trying to block the full contradictory consequences that follow from it is to hide the full spectrum of properties that Christ exemplifies – and that Christians need Christ to exemplify. A full understanding of Christ's contradictory being may be beyond our currently limited epistemic reach; but Christ's reality – by all orthodox lights – is not in any way constrained by our epistemic reach.

Belaboring the point, the practice of christian theology pushes in opposite directions: the truth of Christ's passibility; the falsity of Christ's passibility. And the practice is grounded in the true contradictory theory: one's suffering screams out for the falsity of Christ's having the divine properties, and such falsity is steadfastly there; and one's suffering can also require the truth of Christ's having those properties, and the truth of them is equally steadfastly there. The contradiction is steadfast; its practical import – with respect to what the practicing Christian invokes, leans upon, needs, or so on – can be very much time- and context-relative. The contradictory truth is not blinking from moment to moment (true now, false later, true after that, false after that); it is there, forever and always. But the needs of the practicing Christian, turning in prayer, are often 'blinking' between the need for a genuine Human ('just like me in all limitations'), and the need for a genuine God ('so very much unlike me in the awesome absence of limitations'). And, of course, there may be many moments in practice when both contradictory truths are needed at the same time. (Some versions of 'mystic' traditions in christian practice make vivid illustrations of these sorts of context – not that this chapter or book is in any way within such traditions.)

The details of practical (contradictory) theology are complicated and demand their own book-length treatment. What is clear and easy to state concisely is that Contradictory Christology – or, more generally, a contradictory christian theology – is not a theory without practical upshot.

4.5.6 Not theology

The proposed theory is not theology. Theologians need not master the technical tools of contemporary logic in order to give the true theory of Christ – the true christology – or a true theory of any other theological phenomenon. But the proposed theory – the proposed contradictory christology – requires a mastery of just such technical logic.[49]

Reply. A full-on mastery of logic is not required; but basic competence in logic and its role is required. The viability of any christology – not just that of Contradictory Christology – relies on logic itself, on the logical consequence relation at the bottom of all consequence relations for our true theories (including our true theory of God). Of course, that theology is not about logic is absolutely clear and equally true. But theology needn't be about logic in order for logic to be of fundamental importance in the true theology. Theology relies on logic; and theologians need to be aware of logic's constraints – and, more to the present discussion, logic's space of possibilities.

---

[49] Compare debates over the importance of analytic theology (Crisp and Rea, 2009).

4.5.7 Theological promiscuity

McCall (2019) raises a serious concern about the knock-on effects of Contradictory Christology, even with its conservative account of the source of contradictions in theology (viz., the incarnation):

> It is not hard to imagine a theologian being convinced by Beall and then saying, 'Cool, I no longer need to worry about avoiding contradictions.' Beall might remonstrate with 'No, you theologians should not seek out contradiction!' .... But the theologian's response is quick: 'look, we don't have to seek them out – they are all over the place and come looking for us. They are unavoidable. The good news now is that we don't need to worry about them.'   (McCall, 2019)

How to reply?

Reply. Let me be clear that I defer to McCall's sense of the general proclivities of contemporary theologians. My experience with systematic theologians does not raise the worry that McCall carries; but I gather from McCall's expressed concern that my experience is based on non-representative samples. The question remains: how to respond?

McCall acknowledges that one who advances a theological position cannot control the use to which it will be put by other theologians. Still, his concern reflects the need to be even clearer about the irresponsibility involved in making the leap from some true theological contradictions to many. The imagined response, per McCall's passage above, is that such a so-called leap is in fact very well warranted by the apparent ubiquity of contradictions in theology – from God's too-heavy stone to the core Trinitarian doctrine to God's contradictory knowledge of the claim 'God cannot know this sentence' to so much more. Far from a paucity of apparent contradictions, theology is a cacophonous carousel of core contradictory creeds.

No it isn't. That's my reply: no, theology is plainly contradictory at just one core point – the incarnation. Yes, the omni-god problems need to be addressed, but the only point at which apparently contradictory predicates are explicitly attributed in core theology is Christ's two-natured being – as the fundamental problem attests.[50] The would-be contradiction involved

---

[50] Note that gappy responses to the standard omni-god problems are available where no such gappy solution is available to the apparent contradiction of Christ – inasmuch as the

in God's omni-properties are fairly downstream, whereas the apparent contradiction of Christ's 2-natured being hits the moment one looks at the water. Similarly with the trinity, which is a core axiom of christian theology but which carries the hint of contradiction only if one thinks – for what reason? – that the identity relation involved in the axiom is an equivalence relation (or sanctions substitutivity of 'identicals' so understood)? One reason to think as much is to think that logic itself provides an identity relation which is common throughout all true theories, and that that (alleged) relation is an equivalence relation or at least sanctions substitutivity of 'identicals'. By my lights, that's a mistaken view. But even if such a view were correct, there's no good reason, as far as I can tell, to think that the identity relation involved in the Trinitarian axiom is the relation that logic itself (supposedly) supplies to all true theories.[51]

4.5.8 Direct doctrinal guidance?

McCall (2019) raises a concern for the application of Contradictory Christology to matters of ecumenical doctrine and/or practice:

> A fourth and final question is more directly practical and even pastoral in nature . . . . The question is: how is the account [of a contradictory theology] drawn here to offer helpful practical guidance for Christian communities if it is affirmed and applied more broadly?   (McCall, 2019)

Elaborating on the question McCall writes:

> Doctrine plays important roles in the formation of the community of faith and in the formation of character and the virtues within that faith community. [McCall cites Ellen T. Charry's work (Charry, 1997) as an example.] Will the acceptance of contradictions (in this case of the doctrine

---

fundamental-problem predicates are definitive (axiomatic) of Christ, and so can be gappy only at the cost of heresy. (See, e.g., McCall's echoing of Coakley about the role of the creeds in constraining what true christian theology *must* contain.)

[51] Van Inwagen's pioneering paper on so-called relative identity relations (van Inwagen, 1988) is in keeping with my view of identity relations in theories: the theorist needs to supply her identity relation, which mightn't be an equivalence relation, or mightn't validate (by the lights of the theory's entailment relation) substitution of 'identicals'. See too the earlier work of Martinich (1978).

of the incarnation, at the very heart of the Christian fath, but potentially more broadly as well) actually strengthen the faith of the faithful and assist ecclesial communities in the important work in moral and spiritual formation? Or might it bring harm?   (McCall, 2019)

Illustrating some potential harm that a contradictory theology – indeed, Contradictory Christology (viz., 'at the very heart of the Christian faith') – may carry, McCall presents a scenario in which Catholic leaders assemble top-shelf scholars to evaluate the ordination of women in the priesthood. Lacking no resources accessible to humans, and lacking no time to figure out the issue, the given leaders come to the following position: namely, that both of the statements

- It is true that ordination should be open to women.
- It is false that ordination should be open to women.

enjoy seemingly sound theological arguments. But since sound arguments have true conclusions the sound arguments for both (contradictory) conclusions jointly (logically) entail a contradiction. What to do? A scholar in the gathering points to the fact that logic itself, being suitably subclassical per §2, doesn't rule out the veridicality of the given appearance. Pending some special reason to reject the strong appearance of soundness in both cases, the gathering of scholars and church leaders proffers a unanimous statement to the effect that the given contradiction is true; and the Catholic church in turn declares the matter to be fact (dropping the modal 'should' to the actual 'is'):

- It is true that ordination is open to women.
- It is false that ordination is open to women.

Catholics are thereby required to abide by the moral and ecclesiastical obligations that follow from the truth of both conjuncts.

The point of McCall's scenario is to highlight what he perceives as potential harm flowing from a contradictory theology into the moral obligations of a church (both leaders and laity). How to reply?

Reply. By way of reply, I first note that there's no requirement in Contradictory Christology that any other facet of the true theology – except that which follows directly from the contradiction who is Christ – be contradictory. Accordingly, McCall's scenario is indeed hypothetical, lest any reader should think otherwise. (And to be doubly clear: McCall nowhere suggests that Contradictory Christology requires further contradictions; he only rightly says that it may.)

One question raised by McCall's scenario is whether it's possible. Clearly, the scenario is logically possible; but that's saying little. Moreover, as far as I know, the scenario is theologically possible. One might wonder, though, whether there's some physical impossibility that gets in the way. For example, it's physically (or cognitively or the like) impossible, I believe, to both accept and simultaneously reject the truth of some claim A.[52] It might be that being a priest requires that one accept some claim A while being a non-priest requires that one reject the very same claim A. (I can't think of such a requirement, but for purposes of example imagine that the priesthood demands 'self-reflection' of its priests in such a way that the priest must, on pain of excommunication, accept that they themselves are priests – accept the claim *I am a priest*.) In this case, there's good reason to reject the physical (or cognitive or the like) possibility of McCall's scenario. Whether, then, McCall's scenario is possible in relevant respects turns on further details of the case.

Grant, for discussion, that the scenario is possible in relevant respects. Focus, as is McCall's intended target, on the upshot for the church and its obligations. (I say 'church' rather than 'Church' because McCall's scenario needn't be tied just to one particular tradition such as the Catholic Church.) What guidance should – can – be given by way of carrying out the obligations of the given contradiction concerning ordination? Truly, I do not know. I think that it's a very remote possibility – if, as we're assuming for discussion, a relevant possibility it be – that the church in its wisdom should arrive at such a position. After all, ordination has a very, very direct practical arm to it; and without having some sense of how the practical arm is to function in the final truth about ordination, it is unlikely that top-shelf church leaders will conclude that they've reached the final truth.

None of this is to say that moral dilemmas (even theologically driven moral dilemmas) – namely, moral obligations to do what you cannot relevantly possibly do – refute the truth of the moral claims that result in such dilemmas; they don't. My point about McCall's scenario is that it's at least

---

[52] I'm not alone. Many theorists who either think that there are true glutty theories or think that there are true gappy theories or, like me, think that there are both sorts of such theories, reject that one can simultaneously accept and reject a claim A, even though the glut theorists require, for some A, acceptance of both A and its negation $\neg A$ while the gap theorists require, for some A, rejection of both A and its negation $\neg A$ (Beall, 2009; Field, 2008; Priest, 2006).

implausible that the leaders would unanimously agree that the truth about such an important practical matter results in the obvious dilemma – namely, to both ordain and not ordain women. Does logical space allow it? Yes. Does the space of theological possibility allow it? We're assuming as much, at least for discussion. But does the given scenario reflect a likely practical issue for Contradictory Christianity – as the wider view of which Contradictory Christology is a part? I don't see it.

5

Measured against alternative views

This chapter compares the proposed christology (theology, generally) against a few salient alternatives. The chapter is not in any sense exhaustive; it covers only a few directions of proposed responses to the apparent contradiction of Christ – to the so-called fundamental 'problem' of christology – and focuses only on ones that aim to be both Chalcedon-constrained and in keeping with the standard view of logical consequence. Moreover, since target views are advanced in large works by leaders in the field – works that are easily accessible and speak clearly on differences in detail – the aim of this chapter is to give big-picture sketches of key strategies, leaving references to handle details of individual accounts. The big-picture sketches convey just enough to highlight what I take to be inadequacies of the approaches vis-à-vis Contradictory Christology.

5.1 From incarnation to contradiction

Before turning to the main (consistency-questing) strategies, I briefly rehearse the fundamental problem.

The Council of Chalcedon 451, in response to longstanding quests for consistency (e.g., lingering ideas from Arius, Apollinaris, Nestorius, Eutyches, and others), stamped a fair-dinkum chock-full – 100%-divine and 100%-human – account of the incarnation: Christ is *fully divine* and *fully human*, not mostly human and in-part divine, not mostly divine and in-part human, and not some other hybrid combination of divinity and humanity. Given standard conceptions of divinity and humanity (i.e., of divine nature and human nature), each informed in turn by revelation and, respectively, biology, Chalcedon's account hits a familiar problem, namely, what Richard Cross famously dubbed 'the fundamental problem [of the incarnation]' (Cross, 2011, p. 453). The problem, in short, is that the given chock-full

The Contradictory Christ. Jc Beall, Oxford University Press (2021). © Jc Beall.
DOI: 10.1093/oso/9780198852360.003.0005

account, combined with said classical conceptions, leads to contradiction. Example:

1. Christ is divine. [Rationale: per Chalcedon.]
2. Christ is human. [Rationale: per Chalcedon.]
3. Christ is immutable. [Rationale: 1, entailed by divine nature.]
4. Christ is mutable. [Rationale: 2, entailed by human nature.]
5. It's true that Christ is mutable. [Rationale: 4, truth-operator entailment.]
6. It's false that Christ is mutable. [Rationale: 3, entailment from 'im-'.]
7. It's true that Christ is mutable and it's false that Christ is mutable. [Rationale: 5–6, logic.]

Likewise, mutatis mutandis, for im-/passibility, im-/peccability, im-/materiality, and so on for the many pairs of properties either entailed by the two natures (viz., divine and human) or otherwise affirmed of Christ in Chalcedon 451 and, generally, in 'historic christian orthodoxy', to use a term sometimes used to record historic unity of christian doctrine among salient traditions (viz., Catholic, Orthodox, and Protestant).

5.2 Standard routes towards consistency

Because the incarnation is central to the very foundation of christian theory, the fundamental problem demands a response. The dominant strategy is a quest to consistentize Christ, to give a logically consistent account of the incarnate God. The quest for consistency aims to explain how the apparent contradiction of Christ – the contradiction apparently entailed by Christ's two natures – is merely apparent, to somehow 'eke out' consistency (Coakley, 2002) from the demands of, as above, full-on divinity and full-on humanity – demands that lead to the contradiction as above.

The most influential map of the quest for consistency is that of Cross (2011).[1] Cross' succinct and, at the time, fairly exhaustive map charts the main strategies in the longstanding quest to consistentize Christ. Except for adding an explicit meaning-change option (which is compatible with Cross'

---

[1] Other prominent discussions of the problem are many, including recently that of Adams (2006), Crisp (2007, 2009), McCall (2015), Stump (2003), Morris (1986), Swinburne (1994), Anderson (2007), Pawl (2016, 2020), Leftow (2002), Gorman (2016), and many others.

discussion) and an epistemic-mystery option, I follow the Cross map here, although my presentation should not be read back into Cross' discussion.

5.3 QUA-device accounts

QUA-device strategies are well-known, and their problems are equally well-known.[2] Here, 'Christ is mutable' and/or 'Christ is immutable' are shorthand for 'QUA-adorned truths' – namely, 'Christ-qua-human is mutable' or the like, where different strategies put the QUA device in different places. (More on this below.) The error in the given derivation (page 120) is that premises (1) and (2) are insufficiently expressed: the truths involve QUA adornments that undermine the steps to (5).

For present purposes, I simply highlight what I take to be the glaring defects with the most common of the QUA strategies (viz., 1-QUA strategies illustrated below), at least in comparison with the contradictory account.[3]

5.3.1 1-QUA in abstract

The '1-QUA' terminology arises from applying a QUA device (some variation of 'qua this' or 'qua that') in the 1 position of a typical subject–predicate sentence:

- Subject^1 is^2 P^3

where 'P' stands in for some predicate, and the superscripts mark the relevant positions (viz., 1 is subject, 2 is exemplification, and 3 is property). A typical 1-QUA account maintains that a given QUA device applies to the Subject (or 1st) position, modifying the subject term in some way. A typical spelling of 1-QUA in christology looks something like this:

- *Christ qua N is* P

where the target N is either *divine nature* or *human nature*.

---

[2] Senor (2002) gives an influential chart of the grammatical positions of (what I call) QUA devices, and Cross (2002*a*) discusses the large medieval framework for QUA analyses.
[3] Representative discussions of key problems, discussions with which I largely agree, are given by Senor (2002), Cross (2011) and Pawl (2016). For an influential defense of a particular 1-QUA strategy, see Adams 2006, but see Cross 2011 on where Adams' strategy falters.

Terminology: Call a subject-predicate sentence (e.g., 'S is P') 'QUA-adorned' just if it explicitly uses the target QUA device – in the 1-QUA case, uses 'S-qua-X' (with or without the hyphens) for the subject term; and call the corresponding same subject–predicate sentence 'QUA-*un*adorned' if it does not explicitly use the target QUA device.

5.3.2 The basic 1-QUA strategy

A typical 1-QUA account looks like it rejects the key Chalcedon axioms

C1. Christ is divine.
C2. Christ is human.
C3. There is exactly one person who is Christ.

The 1-QUA approach rejects, on pain of apparent contradiction, the key trio of Chalcedon axioms if left in their unadorned state. As such, the only truths expressed by the axioms are in fact not the QUA-unadorned 'truths' (which are taken to be contradictory) but rather the target QUA-adorned ones: namely,

C1Q. Christ-qua-divine is divine.
C2Q. Christ-qua-human is human.
  C3. There is exactly one person who is Christ.

Of course, instead of outrightly rejecting C1 and C2 in favor of their QUA-adorned siblings (viz., C1Q and C2Q) the 1-QUA strategy may instead affirm C1 and C2 in their unadorned states but reject the usual entailments *as usually given* – namely, the QUA-*un*adorned entailments (e.g., that Christ is immutable and mutable, etc.). The idea here is that, for example, C1 is true – no need for a QUA adornment to express its truth – but the usual *QUA-unadorned* fact entailed by C1, namely,

Ci. Christ is immutable (impassible, impeccable, etc.)

is only *apparently* a fact; the genuine fact entailed by C1 is not Ci but rather the *QUA-adorned*

CiQ. Christ-qua-divine is immutable (impassible, impeccable, etc.)

and, similarly, for the corresponding 'fact' entailed by C2, namely,

CmQ. Christ-qua-human is mutable (passible, peccable, etc.).

Either way, the 1-QUA strategy looks for a consistent account of Christ by adorning christology with otherwise hidden adornments.[4]

There are two intimately related problems with the usual 1-QUA accounts, at least as compared with Contradictory Christology. Take the problems in turn (but note, again, that they are closely related).

5.3.3 Problem 1: Loss of simplicity via multiplication of subjects

Adding QUA adornments, like so many consistency-quest strategies, is a stable route towards a consistent christology that contains both C1 and C2. But one wonders why we're now talking about these other two subjects – namely, *Christ-qua-divine* and *Christ-qua-human* – when our principal focus was supposed to be Christ. One wonders why we're now multiplying subjects beyond Christ himself.

The quest for consistency, on the 1-QUA account, pushes away from a simple picture of Christ as the principal exemplification of humanity and divinity (and all that's thereby entailed) and towards a complex multiplication of subjects.

5.3.4 Problem 2: Shifting the principal subject

1-QUA explains the would-be consistency of the target axioms (viz., C1 and C2) by multiplying entities into what, compared with the QUA-free picture, is not only baroque or complex; it shifts the principal subject matter of christology away from Christ – the person who is God, the same person who hung on the cross covered in dirt, blood, and aspersions. How did God hang on the cross?

- The QUA-*ful* answer: he-qua-human hung on the cross.
- The QUA-*free* answer: he was human; he hung on the cross.

---

[4] The 2-QUA and 3-QUA strategies are the same except for where the adornments go (Cross, 2002*a*, 2011; Pawl, 2016), as is the so-called 0-QUA strategy (Beall and Henderson, 2019).

These two answers are not equivalent on the QUA account: if they were, Christ-qua-human is identical to Christ, in which case the elaborate edifice collapses back into contradiction. The QUA-free answer keeps the focus squarely on Christ; the QUA-ful answer shifts the focus to other subjects (viz., 'Christ-qua-human').

Problem 1, as above, is a multiplication of subjects and the resulting complexity thereby incurred. Problem 2 – intimately tied to Problem 1 – is a shifting of focus. In an effort to achieve a consistent account of Christ the 1-QUA view multiplies entities and then shifts the principal subject from Christ to said entities. Christ, in the end, is only derivatively the bearer of divine and human properties; the principal subjects of these properties are Christ-qua-divine and Christ-qua-human. In a very plain sense, one looks to 'save Christ' from inconsistency by talking about other distinct subjects that don't bear the contrary properties that Christ has long been thought to bear – namely, either divinity and humanity or the standard properties entailed therefrom.

Some might see such remarks as a contentious characterization of the situation. I do not. The whole point of the Chalcedon account, as I see it, is to characterize Christ as exactly one person who is both divine and human, one person who has all properties characteristic of divine beings and human beings. Given the apparent contradiction of a divine person who is human (and all that that entails) the 1-QUA account shifts the subject from that person – namely, Christ – to two other entities, namely, Christ-qua-divine and Christ-qua-human. What are these other principal players? The natural answer is that they are 'natures'. But now the longstanding issue: if the natures are 'abstract' (say, modeled as sets of properties) then it's crystal clear that the natures are merely *explaining* why Christ – the principal subject – exemplifies the full set of divine and human properties; and so, contrary to my foregoing remarks, there is no genuine multiplication of subjects and subsequent shifting of subjects. That's good. On the other hand, on this 'abstract' approach to *Christ-qua-N*, it is no longer clear how the target contradiction is avoided. (After all, if saying that Christ-qua-divine is immutable is to say that Christ *because he exemplifies the divine nature* is immutable, then we're back to the fundamental contradiction of Christ's being immutable and mutable.) Accordingly, to avoid the apparent contradiction of Christ the target natures – the subjects named 'Christ-qua-human' and 'Christ-qua-divine' – are sometimes taken to be 'concrete'. On this view, these subjects are the principal subjects of what we erroneously thought were Christ's properties; but it turns out that Christ enjoys those properties only derivatively; the principal subjects are the various things we're calling 'concrete natures'. Unlike the 'abstract' approach, the apparent contradiction of Christ's would-be properties is avoided because ultimately Christ only has such properties derivatively – by charity, as said in previous chapters. But the cost of avoiding the contradiction in this way is that, contrary to the charge of being contentious, the charge of a multiplication of subjects and shifting of principal subjects is spot on.[5]

5.4 Explicitly compositional accounts

In many ways the compositional accounts are structurally like the 1-QUA strategy except that, in general, they attempt to motivate the strategies with a metaphysical account of parts and wholes or, more neutrally, 'composition' of subjects. Here, the target predicates are again, at least in effect if not in offical letter, *primarily* applied to proper 'parts' (or aspects or elements or whathaveyou) of Christ – in the most general sense of 'parts' – and so only *derivatively* to Christ. Example: Christ's *physical body* is mutable but no divine 'part' of Christ is mutable. Here, the contradiction fails because step (3) in the fundamental-problem derivation (page 120) fails: an object can be mutable in virtue of one of its features (parts, etc.) but immutable in virtue of another – no more inconsistent than 'in-part green' and 'in-part red', applied to one object, are inconsistent.[6]

The part–whole strategies towards consistentizing Christ may be natural – and are very popular – for those on the longstanding quest, and they are intimately tied in natural ways to a variety of QUA strategies, as indicated above. Still, in comparison with Contradictory Christology, such strategies appear to be largely without motivation.

---

[5] Senor (2002) raises at least the spirit of the same shifts-the-principal-subject objection but does so in the letter of Nestorian red flags, a charge that, as Cross (2011) notes, is at least in need of further argument in the face of medieval 'specificative' analyses. My objection is neutral on Nestorianism; it's simply that an account that shifts the principal focus away from Christ – as the principal property bearer of all given divine and all given human properties – is prima facie worse (because prima facie off-topic) than an account that keeps Christ as the fundamental bearer of the given properties.

[6] There is obviously a lot of room to have rival accounts along these lines, depending on notions of 'parts', composition (mereological or otherwise), metaphysics of natures, etc. Pawl (2016, 2019b) explores these issues at great length, developing at least an implicitly compositional but officially non-mereological account, while two influential explicitly compositional accounts are by Stump (2003) and Leftow (2002).

The problem, at least with the contradictory option firmly at hand, is straightforward, and exactly similar to the problem with 1-QUA accounts. The core christian account is exceedingly simple on its surface: Christ is divine and Christ is human. And Christ is a person, and so is a divine person and a human person. Christ is the bearer of all such properties (viz., all those properties entailed by either divinity or humanity) – the primary, fundamental bearer of all such properties. That's the simple and core picture. Deviation from the simple core is motivated if the core carries a substantial problem – if it's rotten, so to speak. But now the question: why reject the core picture? Why complicate the core characterization of Christ with explicit (or even just implicit) talk about two or more other primary bearers of what, on the simple picture, are properties primarily exemplified by Christ? In short: why isn't Christ the fundamental bearer of the extraordinary pool of divine and human properties? Why other things?

The answer is obvious: namely, Christ can't be the primary bearer or fundamental bearer of such properties because – and here's the familiar rub – such properties jointly entail a contradiction. Were Christ the fundamental bearer of all such properties Christ would be contradictory. And that's simply not on, as the compositional strategies reflect. A fundamental commitment to the consistency of Christ drives the explicitly compositional accounts.

The motivation for compositional strategies is just as above: namely, we should reject that Christ is a contradictory being (why?) but, in keeping with Chalcedon's stamp of both full-on divinity and full-on humanity, we must maintain that Christ *somehow* – in *some* way or other – has the properties entailed by divinity and entailed by humanity. And now the compositional account rolls out: namely, just say that Christ's two distinguishing natures are proper parts, one part being the fundamental bearer of divine properties, the other being the fundamental bearer of human properties. Because the proper parts are Christ's proper parts, Christ – as the relevant whole – gets to have all such properties *in part*: Christ is *in-part mutable*, which is to say, Christ has a proper part which (fundamentally etc.) is mutable; Christ is *in-part immutable*, which is to say, Christ has a proper part which (fundamentally etc.) is immutable; and so on. Even though compositional accounts tend not to explicitly use the 'in-part' expression in official accounts, this familiar expression, for all that I can see, is the critical key: there's no contradiction – or even hint of contradiction – because, when properly given, the core christological claims stamped at Chalcedon have an implicit 'in-part' rider.

The loudest question, at least by my lights, is also the obvious one: why not just say so from the start? Why say only

1. Christ is fully divine.
2. Christ is fully human.

when in fact what was meant all along is the very easy-to-state rider claims

1P. Christ is in-part fully divine (i.e., has a fully divine part).
2P. Christ is in-part fully human (i.e., has a fully human part).

The standard entailments from (1) are vastly different from those of 1P, and likewise for (2) and 2P. The latter claims are not even remotely (or even prima facie weakly) puzzling if, as perhaps a default reading would have, the relevant parts – whatever they may be – are not identical. (If they were, then we have the fundamental problem arising all over again for the puzzling divine–human part.) The former claims are prima facie (and even historically) deeply puzzling because they seem to entail a contradiction. (Witness: the fundamental problem.)

I take (1) and (2) to be the key claims, not 1P or 2P. Compositional strategies appear to make 1P and 2P the key christological claims.

The problem with compositional strategies, at least in comparison with the contradictory account, is not only in the apparent switch from (1) and (2) to 1P and 2P; it's also the requirement, riding right on the surface of such accounts, of fairly substantial metaphysics. This too is the same issue raised elsewhere (e.g., §3), but it is worth flagging again. Contradictory Christology, which makes perfectly good sense of the core claims (1) and (2) in their powerful simplicity, is neutral with respect to the true theory of metaphysics, including the true metaphysics of parts and wholes, the true metaphysics of persons, and more. The viability and indeed truth of the contradictory account are independent from the difficult metaphysics of persons, parts, and their combinations. While there is a full and true metaphysics of parts and wholes (and, of course, their relation, if any, to persons and their 'makeup'), and while the truth may well be per some compositional account of Christ or other, the would-be consistency of Christ shouldn't be staked on such an account, at least in the absence of clear revelation or ecumenical decree on the true metaphysics, or simply clear discovery of the true metaphysics. It'd be one matter were the true metaphysics to be revealed in some as yet unknown way, or were to be officially stamped by the church universal; however, no such revelation or stamp has been delivered, at least as far as I can see.

In the end, compositional strategies towards a consistent account of Christ appear to be both under-motivated and overly biased, at least in comparison with Contradictory Christology. The under-motivated status starts from scratch: why complicate the powerful simplicity of (1) and (2) when their only alleged 'problem' is the consequence that Christ is a contradictory being? The overly-biased status is the requisite metaphysical filling that cannot but accompany such a strategy. There's nothing whatsoever wrong with finding the true metaphysics; that project should continue – just as the project of finding the true physics, true biology, and so on should continue. But to stake the truth of Christ on such projects, at least when the 'problem' has a ready and simple solution, appears to stake too much. Again, were there some very good reason to reject the simpler contradictory solution, there'd thereby be increased motivation for the compositional accounts.

5.5   Explicit meaning-changing accounts

Here, among many other in-principle options, there are two salient directions, one that Cross (2011) calls 'restriction', which aims specifically at the standard meanings of 'divine' or 'human', and one that retains (in some sense) the standard meanings of 'divine' and 'human' while explicitly switching, in ways explained below, the meanings (viz., satisfaction conditions) of predicates entailed by 'divine' and 'human'. In ways that are illustrated below, and for lack of better terms, I call the former strategy *upstream changes* and the latter *downstream changes*, although tags of 'stage 1' and 'stage 2' might be equally useful.

While the upstream and downstream strategies are different in both motivation and implementation, my evaluation of both strategies points to roughly the same problem, at least in comparison with the contradictory account I'm advancing. This is not in any way to suggest that the two strategies are on par in all respects; they're not. But highlighting their similar problems – at least vis-à-vis Contradictory Christology – suffices for present purposes.

Terminology. In what follows, I employ familiar talk of *predicate entailment*. Let P and P' be predicates in a given theory T, and let T-entailment be T's consequence relation (per §2). Predicate entailment (relative to theory T etc.) is understood thus: P *T-entails* P' if and only if an object's satisfying P T-entails its satisfying P'.

Terminology generalized. Similarly, generalizing predicate-predicate entailment to a predicate's *T-entailing a set of predicates* (so, generalizing to predicate-set entailment), let us say that a predicate P *T-entails a set S of predicates* iff P T-entails each predicate in S.[7] This suffices for background terminology.

5.5.1 Upstream meaning changes: 'divine' and 'human'

Start with the abstract picture. Suppose that a predicate P entails a set S of predicates, say, $S = \{P_1, P_2, \ldots, P_n\}$.[8] An *upstream* meaning change switches from P itself to some restricted predicate P' where P' entails only a *proper subset* of S.[9] The key here is that there's no downstream change (so to speak) in the satisfaction conditions (i.e., the meanings) of *predicates in S itself* (e.g., 'immutable' and 'mutable' mean what they standardly mean); the change is rather in the 'upstream' predicate P itself, weakening the entailments to only a proper subset of S.[10] This 'upstream' change from P to P' opens the following option: an object that satisfies P satisfies each and every element of S, but an object satisfying only (the weaker) P' need satisfy only a proper subset of S.

Turning to the target application, upstream accounts change either 'divine' or 'human' (or both) to some restricted cousin.[11] With an eye on the target derivation on page 120, and just picking 'divine' (versus 'human') for illustration, the strategy changes the meaning of 'divine' to '⋆-divine', which,

---

[7] This is not so-called multiple-conclusion entailment. T-entailment of a set of predicates requires entailment of all elements in the entailed set, as above.

[8] Strictly speaking, what we're entertaining is some theory T according to which P T-entails each element of S, but for convenience I drop the explicit reference to T except where confusion may arise.

[9] Terminology: a set X is a *subset* of a set Y iff every element of X is an element of Y. (Therefore, every set X is a subset of itself.) Sets X and Y are *identical* iff X is a subset of Y and Y is a subset of X. (Therefore, X and Y are identical sets iff there's no difference in their respective elements.) Finally, a set X is a *proper subset* of a set Y iff X is a subset of Y but X is not identical to Y. (Therefore, given said identity conditions on sets, if X is a *proper subset* of Y then every element of X is in Y but there's at least one element of Y which is not in X.)

[10] One can accordingly also think of this as a change in the entailment relation that defines P, one relation going from P to S, the new one going from P to S', where S' is a proper subset of S. But I'll just speak of changing P itself to some cousin P' – some 'restricted' cousin, per Cross' terminology (2011) – that entails a proper subset of the predicates that P entails.

[11] In salient work in this direction, restrictions are generally placed on 'human', but, as discussion in the area reflects, it is difficult to see how changes only to one of the two upstream predicates is sustainable without upending the theological tradition that motivates it. Detailed discussion is given by Morris (1986), Swinburne (1994), Cross (2011), Gorman (2016), and references in the given works.

unlike 'divine', fails to entail 'immutable'. In material terms, the property of being ★-divine (pronounce: star divine), unlike that of being divine – unlike, that is, the property standardly expressed by 'divine' – does not involve immutability: ★-divine beings can change, but divine beings (if any there be on the upstream account) cannot. Likewise, mutatis mutandis, for im-/passible, im-/peccable, in-/visible, and perhaps similarly for temporal or omni- properties, or even im-/perfect and/or more. Accordingly, ★-divine beings appear not to be perfect in the way that divine beings are standardly taken to be perfect, since perfect beings can't change from perfection to anything less or more than perfection. Weaken the direct entailments of 'divinity' and one thereby has a divine (or, more precisely, ★-divine) being whose 'divinity' is clearly weaker than that of a would-be divine being where 'divine' has its standard entailments running full stream. And that's the point of upstream meaning change: avoid the apparent contradiction of Christ by diminishing the upstream notions of divinity or humanity or both.

On an upstream meaning-change strategy the fundamental error in the target derivation (page 120) is either the step from (1) to (3) or from (2) to (4) – or, of course, both – depending on which side of the stream one takes. The 'two chock-ful natures' stamped by Chalcedon in (1) and (2) remains true and firmly part of the theory; it's just that the predicates have implicit stars that flag weaker entailments than the standard predicates enjoy. The demands of being 'fully human' and, equally, 'fully divine' are far fewer than what standard stamps portray; the Chalcedon stamp achieves consistency by using lookalikes, by using fainter images of divinity and/or humanity than standard usage implies.

To put an instance of the upstream strategy in a diagram (of sorts),[12] let ⇒ indicate the theory's predicate-entailment relation, so that

$$P \Rightarrow Q$$

is shorthand for the claim that predicate P entails predicate Q, and similarly for predicate-set entailments defined per §5.5, namely,

$$P \Rightarrow \{P_1, P_2, \ldots, P_n\}$$

is shorthand for the claim that P entails the given set of predicates. Then the *standard* entailments towards the apparent contradiction of Christ are E1–E4 (focusing here just on the example of im-/mutability):

---

[12] Note well: this is just an instance of the upstream strategy; it's not intended to be the paradigm example of the strategy.

E1. 'divine' ⇒ 'immutable'.

and the downstream truth that

E2. 'immutable' ⇒ 'unchanging'.

in addition to the transitivity of the given entailments, namely,

E3. 'divine' ⇒ 'unchanging'.

and, in turn,

E4. 'unchanging' ⇒ 'doesn't change'.

On standard usage, Christ's being divine entails that Christ is unchanging (or at least unchangeable). Likewise, mutatis mutandis, for Christ's being human entailing the falsity of Christ's being unchanging (or at least the falsity of Christ's being unchangeable).

Facing the contradiction from Christ's being divine and human, the *upstream* strategy stops and pivots at scratch: *replace* E1 – and do likewise for all occurrences of 'divinity' in the theory, including especially core premises (1) and (2) in the target derivation (page 120). By way of replacement, the upstream strategy puts its 'restricted' notion of divinity in place, namely, ⋆-divinity, a property that can be had *without contradiction* by beings who change. Whatever its other entailments may be, the new predicate '⋆-divine' fails to entail immutability:

E5. '⋆-divine' ⇏ 'immutable'.

Since, according to the new theory, Christ is only ⋆-divine the march towards the otherwise apparent contradiction of Christ is arrested.

5.5.2 Downstream meaning changes: 'immutable' and 'mutable' etc.

Downstream accounts differ from upstream accounts in their point of entry – the place at which explicit meaning change occurs. A key motivation for downstream accounts is the thought that weakening the divinity of Christ – of God – to some starred notion with fewer than the standard entailments is more intrusive or damaging to the theological theory than forcing meaning changes elsewhere. A less intrusive route leaves 'divine' and 'human' alone (in some sense) and weakens the entailments elsewhere. Upstream meaning-change accounts change the direct entailments of the upstream notion (e.g., restrict the set of predicates directly entailed by the given upstream notion); *downstream* meaning-change accounts change the entailments *of* the (direct) entailments of the upstream notion. That's the basic difference.

Return to the abstract picture from above (see §5.5.1). Suppose, again, that a predicate P entails a set S of predicates, say, $S = \{P_1, P_2, \ldots, P_n\}$. A *downstream* account aims to retain P's standard meaning by 'retaining' (in some sense) the entailment from P to S; the explicit change occurs not directly in the satisfaction conditions governing P but rather in the 'downstream' elements of S itself. In short, a downstream account changes the meanings – the satisfaction conditions – of at least some of the elements P_i in S. (For simplicity, I focus only on the case of changing all elements P_i in S.) The picture, in abstract, changes from $S = \{P_1, P_2, \ldots, P_n\}$, where S is entailed by P on standard meanings, to $S' = \{P'_1, P'_2, \ldots, P'_n\}$, where P'_1, P'_2, and so on, each has a different meaning from its standard counterparts in S. This 'downstream' change from S to S' allows for the option of satisfying the upstream P without thereby satisfying the entailments *of* the entailments of P.[13]

A concrete illustration, following the implementation of Pawl (2016), is useful.[14] Focusing here on *mutability* and *immutability* as a representative pair, Pawl's change-the-meaning recipe runs as follows.

- Standard usage:

  » s is *mutable* iff s is able to change.
  » s is *immutable* iff it's false that s is mutable.

---

[13] One can now easily see why it's awkward to claim, without shudder quotes, that the downstream strategy 'retains' the standard meaning of upstream P. Still, the difference in the explicit meaning-change strategies is clear enough at least with respect to their respective targets of explicit change.

[14] This should not be read as an exposition of Pawl's position; the aim is to illustrate the downstream strategy by illustrating one leading way in which it has been implemented. My presentation is written for current discussion; its aim is not to convey the exact details of Pawl's account. Those details are readily available in Pawl's work (2016, 2019b).

The key ingredient in the recipe is a downstream change of meanings, one deriving from (piggybacking on) the standard usage:[15]

- Starred usage:

  » *s* is ★-*mutable* iff *s* has a 'concrete nature' which is mutable.
  » *s* is ★-*immutable* iff *s* has a 'concrete nature' which is immutable.

This recipe is generalized to all fundamental-problem predicates. It's clear that, as above, changing the satisfaction conditions from the standard conditions to the starred conditions weakens the downstream consequences. And that's the point of the downstream (similarly, upstream) strategies: weaken the consequences so as to avoid the apparent contradiction of Christ.

Though details of implementation can differ, the downstream strategy is ultimately the same as the upstream: weaken the entailments *of* the entailments of 'divine' (ditto 'human') and one can thereby have a 'divine' being whose would-be divinity is clearly weaker – at least downstream – than standard entailments otherwise reflect.

The downstream account deviates from the upstream account by not starring 'divine'. Instead, as above, the stars attach to 'immutability' and the like. But the stars can't just stop there; they need to go everywhere downstream – all the way down to 'changing' and 'unchanging' and the like. To see this, consider the diagram of entailments E1-E4 above (page 131). The downstream strategy replaces E1 in favor of

E6. 'divine' $\Rightarrow$ '★-immutable'.

In turn, the downstream strategy takes a *star-it-all* approach to E2 and the rest:

E7. '★-immutable' $\Rightarrow$ '★-unchanging'

---

[15] Reference to 'concrete natures' in the following 'starred' conditions reflects a substantial metaphysical commitment on the implementation advanced by Pawl's downstream strategy. I flag it because it's a significant feature of the approach, but not one on which I comment further here. (Though Pawl explicitly rejects mereological accounts, his downstream strategy – in particular, the starred satisfaction conditions above – is motivated by compositional considerations involving the 'parts' of Christ in the very broadest sense of the term, a sense covering 'aspects' of Christ, properties of Christ, and so on.)

where, following the general downstream strategy of Pawl (2016, 2019*b*) to its implicit end, one has

- Starred usage:

  » *s* ⋆-*changes* iff *s* has a 'concrete nature' which changes.
  » *s* is ⋆-*unchanging* iff *s* has a 'concrete nature' which is unchanging.

This results in a full-on change of meaning everywhere downstream from – but not including – 'divine' and 'human', leaving Christ as one who is neither mutable nor immutable (more on which below) but instead simply ⋆-mutable and ⋆-immutable, and in turn as one who ⋆-changes and is ⋆-unchanging, and so on. The starred predicates are weaker than the un-starred ones, and Christ's divinity and humanity are in that respect weaker than standard usage suggests. Such weakness is the price – indeed, the aim – of avoiding the otherwise contradictory properties of Christ.

5.5.3 Evaluation: meaning-change strategies

There are lots of details-based issues that arise for meaning-change strategies, but as my aim is to keep details at a minimum and focus on the big picture, my evaluation highlights only a few large-scale items, all measured in comparison with Contradictory Christology.

5.5.3.1 Why reject the unstarred theory?
Meaning change is a rejection of the standard theory – a rejection of the standard christology.[16] Meaning change is also a last resort, an option taken only when there are no other viable candidates for the truth. But, as I've argued in this book, the contradictory account accommodates the full divinity of Christ and, equally, the full humanity of Christ, and it does so upstream, downstream, and without in any way depleting or diverting the

---

[16] If the claim were that the theory is overly indeterminate, then this is a different position whereby either one doesn't know what the theory is – in which case, affirming 'it' is awkward at best and irresponsible at worst – or one knows what the theory is but claims that its terms are semantically defective or vague or the like, in which case, again, presumably one is not in position to recognize that the theory entails a contradiction, or in any event one should work rather on the general issue of semantically defective discourse and simply apply the truth from there to christology. Either way, this sort of invocation of indeterminacy is very different from the extant meaning-change strategies, and I set it aside.

stream. Since accommodation of both the full divinity and full humanity of Christ is precisely what the meaning-change accounts are after, the last-resort meaning-change strategy need not be swum.

Of course, actual meaning-change strategists may claim that the *logical consistency* – the *freedom from contradiction* – is a weightier desideratum on the true christology than one that maintains the standard meanings of the theory (i.e., the christology). But this strikes me as in dire need of warrant, at least in the face of a viable contradictory account. There is no revelation that dictates that logical consequence is 'explosive' (i.e., that an arbitrary contradiction logically entails every sentence), let alone that it's per the mainstream account. Moreover, to my knowledge, the catholic church (small 'c'), constrained at least by Chalcedon 451, is not officially obligated to accept an explosive account of logical consequence any more than it's obligated to accept such and so theory of biology, of sets, of properties, of tractors, of quarks, or so on. On what, then, does the dogmatic commitment to the explosiveness of logical consequence rest? Pending a good answer, it's difficult to see why the last-resort option of meaning changes is motivated in the face of an account that preserves the standard meanings, preserves the full-on humanity and full-on divinity (and not by substituting weaker notions), and does so up, down, and throughout the christology.

5.5.3.2 Why not 'structural' change over key semantic change?
Furthermore, suppose that, contrary to appearances, there's some very good reason to reject the contradictory account, and the last-resort strategy of meaning change is the remaining option. Well, there are meaning changes and there are meaning changes; the pressing question concerns the best target of terminological change. Is changing the set of key fundamental terms – the terms that are traditionally taken (and officially used in official doctrinal stamps) – the best option? By my lights, examining (let me say) 'structural' changes in the systematic framework, ones that leave the meanings of core christological predicates (e.g., 'divine', 'immutable', etc.) in place, is a prima facie better first step than to muck with said predicates. Are there any such strategies? I conjecture that there are oodles of unexplored strategies, each aiding those who refuse (for what reason?) to abandon the quest for consistency.

An unexplored change-the-meaning strategy, which may be easier (and more metaphysically neutral) than extant change-the-meaning strategies, changes the standard account of 'definitional conditionals', those conditionals underwriting key definitions (e.g., x is divine *iff-by-definition* such and such). The idea, in a nutshell, is just this: let the biconditionals in the various target definitions fail to detach – that is, fail to satisfy (unrestricted) modus ponens.

** *Parenthetical (technical) note.* (This technical note can be skipped without loss by any readers unfamiliar with so-called normal modal logic.) An easy but crude way to model the running idea: take a standard modal setting and introduce a definitional-conditional connective $\leadsto$ with the following conditions:

- $A \leadsto B$ is true-at-world-w iff there's no $R^{\leadsto}$-accessible world at which A is true but B untrue.
- Allow but *do not require* that $R^{\leadsto}$ is reflexive. (This allows for a world whereat A is true and B untrue but the given world isn't accessible via $R^{\leadsto}$ to itself.)

Define consequence per usual: A entails (or has as a consequence) B iff there's no world of any model at which A is true but B untrue. Now – for the easiest but crudest example – consider a world of some model that stands in the access relation $R^{\leadsto}$ to no worlds in the model, and just let A be true there, B be untrue there. By the truth-at-world conditions for $\leadsto$ above, $A \leadsto B$ is true there too. The idea, then, is to use something like $\leadsto$ as the conditional involved in theology's key definitions driving the fundamental contradictions. *End note.* **

    This unexplored idea, as far as I can see (and, of course, details will tell), is a potentially simpler approach to consistentizing Christ than standard change-the-meaning options that target critical fundamental theological terms. Moreover, that 'definitional conditionals' don't unrestrictedly detach is hardly new; it has roots in fields independent from theology. For example, though it pursues a very different line, the work of Gupta and Belnap (1993) in so-called revision-theoretic frameworks allows for definitional conditionals that behave differently from the usual (say) material conditional or other standard conditionals.

5.6 Identity-relation accounts

Here, the idea is that the consistency of Christ is achieved via theory-specific identity relations. The chief implementation of this idea (on which I focus) is the so-called relative-identity strategy.

The relative-identity strategy, at least with respect to christology (my focus throughout), is more the promise of a strategy than a strategy. The promise rests on the fact that if the identity relation(s) in core christological claims have features that differ from those reflected in the standard account of (absolute, non-relative) identity, then, depending on the details governing the given identity relation, the core christological claims can avoid the apparent contradiction of Christ. This is obviously true. Indeed, on a different but theologically related topic, it's fairly clear, I think (see §6), that 'the' relation of identity involved in at least the trinity is not per the standard account; it doesn't sanction intersubstitutability of 'identicals', and, unless 'the' relation is a terrifically large plurality of relations (per the relative-identity ideas discussed below), it is non-transitive.

The promise of so-called relative-identity accounts goes back to the work of Geach (1980), the subsequent exploratory work of Martinich (1978) and, with an explicit focus on christology, the well-known but entirely defensive work of van Inwagen (1994) – defensive in the sense that, as with van Inwagen's earlier work on the topic (viz., van Inwagen 1988), it's explicitly advanced only to show that there are provably consistent ways to represent core christological claims, but not that any of the charted representations adequately capture a well-defined notion of relative identity that is adequate for the true christology.

Because of the still-programmatic status of the relative-identity promise, my aim here is simply to flag a number of observations and comments by way of comparing the promise to that of Contradictory Christology. Towards that end, I focus largely on the defensive work of van Inwagen (1994) because it's generally cited as one of the leading relative-identity candidates.[17]

In salient ways, the relative-identity promise is similar to both the 1-QUA and explicitly compositional strategies in that, ultimately, the contradiction of Christ is rejected in favor of two 'non-identical' subjects of the otherwise contradiction-entailing properties (e.g., passible, impassible, etc.). The salient difference is that instead of rejecting 'Christ is divine' and 'Christ is human' in favor of QUA-adorned claims, and instead of inflating the metaphysics of Christ's would-be part–whole relations, the relative-identity strategy simply points to the peculiar identity relation of christology, a relation that fails to validate standard substitution principles (e.g., from the

---

[17] Jedwab 2015 is perhaps the most exhaustive and up-to-date discussion of specifically relative-identity strategies, but doesn't appear to answer the few core issues I raise here. See too Baber 2015.

'relative-identity' of x and y, together with the fact that predicate G is true of x, it doesn't follow that G is true of y too), and indeed such target relations fail to satisfy reflexivity (viz., not every element of the domain of discourse need be 'relatively identical' to itself). Details on any of the relative-identity accounts remain in the promissory stage, at least as far as I can tell; however, the idea is suggestive enough to make two observations.

5.6.1 Evaluation

At least in one of its most prominent christological implementations (viz., van Inwagen's work), the strategy is explicitly a defensive strategy: namely, 'to show that the doctrine can be stated without formal contradiction' (van Inwagen, 1994, p. 202). Of course, as all of the other strategies show, the quest for a consistent account of Christ can be achieved in many directions, and the relative-identity account is indeed another such direction. What is the promise of the relative-identity idea vis-à-vis Contradictory Christology?

5.6.1.1 May avoid familiar problems but so does the contradictory account

One important positive note is that the relative-identity idea promises to avoid some of the problems of the other approaches: at the very least, it promises to remain as metaphysically neutral as the contradictory account, and also – so far as I can tell – equally as epistemologically neutral as the contradictory account. This is a definite positive if the promise pans out, though not a unique positive in comparison with the contradictory account, which is equally neutral along the given fronts.[18]

---

[18] Rea (2003, 2011) has a very different view on the would-be relative-identity promise of metaphysical neutrality (at least as applicable to the trinity theses), arguing that anti-realist metaphysics invariably follows. Indeed, along different lines, Brower and Rea (2005) argue that a metaphysical approach to at least trinitarian identity relations is required. (Neither Rea nor Brower discuss the application of their account to Christ.) My criticism of the relative-identity strategy, at least van Inwagen's implementation, is in §5.6.1.2; Rea and I seem to agree on the shortcomings of the van Inwagen account; the difference is that Rea thinks (and Brower too) that the solution to apparent contradictions of the trinity rests in finding a metaphysical relation that underwrites a metaphysically rich account of relative identity. My view, as reflected in the exploratory §6, is that the apparent contradictions of the trinity don't obviously drive theology to relative-identity accounts of the trinitarian-identity relation; however, this topic – namely, the trinity – demands a much longer and deeper discussion than the current work can sustain (including the remarks in §6).

Another potential virtue is that, despite the multiplication of subjects (at least if we count per the multitude of posited relative-identity relations), a multiplication common to many of the consistency-seeking strategies, relative-identity ideas might avoid the problem of shifting the focus away from Christ. This is very important. The shifting-the-focus problem arises because on such shifting-subjects approaches Christ *is not identical to* the 'fundamental subjects' of otherwise contradictory properties, the fundamental subjects carrying the weight of Christ's would-be consistency. But on the relative-identity idea, the problematic non-identity between Christ and the given (let me say) 'consistentizing subjects' is not a non-identity. The running idea, whatever else it may involve, can affirm not the 'identity simpliciter' of Christ and the consistentizing subjects (for there is no such 'identity simpliciter' involved on the given idea) but rather a family of relative-identity relations: Christ is identical-sub-god to whatever exemplifies the divine properties of Christ;[19] Christ is identical-sub-human to whatever exemplifies the human properties of Christ. In compositional, 1-QUA, and downstream meaning-change strategies, Christ is not identical to the principal or primary consistentizing subjects of Christ's divine and human properties; if Christ were so identical, consistency would be lost. Not so with the relative-identity idea: the shift-the-subject objection doesn't arise if Christ is in fact 'identical' – or at least identical-sub-X for a variety of would be identity relations X – with the would-be consistentizing subjects of Christ's properties. Like the promise of metaphysical and epistemological neutrality, the promise of avoiding a shift in principal subject is a definite positive, though, again, not in comparison with the contradictory account, which equally avoids such a shift.

Compared with other consistentizing strategies, the relative-identity idea carries genuine promise. But for all the good that the relative-identity idea promises, the promise strikes me as less natural than the contradictory one. There is no question that consistency can (indeed, is) achieved in a theory of Christ underwritten by a variety of non-standard identity relations, including relative-identity relations. That's not the issue – and should not in any way be in any doubt. The question to ask is whether the apparent contradiction of Christ is better explained by the simple truth that Christ is a contradictory being or whether it's better explained by a semi-complicated

---

[19] The 'identical-sub-god' tag is mine, but it flags one among many would-be relations that are supposed to play key roles in relative-identity promises.

(but as yet not fully defined) notion of relative-identity underwriting the key identity theses of true theology.

** *Parenthetical remark.* I do think that one *might* argue from a principle that the trinity and incarnation demand exactly the same 'solutions' inasmuch as they are both 'problems' (if problems they be). The relative-identity thesis in christian theology was born from reflection on the trinity, and then extended to the incarnation. If the contradictory account cannot be equally extended to the trinity then – the argument might go – we're better off going the relative-identity route, just for unity-of-solutions to the problems. Of course, the contradictory account can be extended to the trinity (via a glut-theoretic account of trinitarian identity, which would naturally involve a non-transitive identity relation); however, the critical question is whether the truth of the trinity is as clearly contradictory as the fundamental 'problem' of the incarnation suggests of Christ. By my lights, the answer is open. Further discussion of a glut-theoretic treatment of the trinity is in §6. *End remark.* **

5.6.1.2 What exactly is relative identity? Or what is even sufficient for it?

Nobody at any time should ever doubt that the doctrine of God incarnate can be stated without formal contradiction: one can find formally consistent ways to say just about anything. Where the difficulty arises is in saying what the core christological theses seem to say. And a key question for relative-identity strategies is just that: what is it to say of things in our domain of discourse (of our theory, or even outside of our theories) that they are *relatively identical* or, more clearly, that, for some suitable expression (sortal, so-called count noun, etc.) N, that they are *the same N*? As far as I can tell, this question remains unanswered in any of the proposed christology-driven 'logics of relative identity'.

The most prominent incarnation-driven work along the relative-identity idea (van Inwagen, 1994) is largely silent on exactly what a relative-identity relation formally amounts to. What is given is (enough of) a formal language into which some English (or, at least, theological-English) sentences may be formally represented, though what makes the representations good or adequate formal representations turns on details that are missing. In particular, there's insufficient information governing the key notion of relative-identity (i.e., the family of so-called relative-identity predicates in the language). What's missing is at least a sufficient condition for such claims.

There's no question that one can find formal representations of theological axioms (so to speak) in a formal relative-identity language and, in turn, prove that no formal contradiction is derivable in the system from elementary axioms (so to speak). This can and has been done (van Inwagen, 1994).[20] But even by the lights of leading theorists such as van Inwagen (1994), to do just that is to do nothing more than show that there is a formal representation that can be constrained so as not to deliver the apparent contradictions of Christ:[21]

> It is time now to show that the whole set of sentences we have endorsed is consistent – that no contradiction [i.e., sentence of the form !A] can be deduced from its members by RI-logic [which is the 'logic of relative identity' advanced]. It will not be surprising if this is so, for the deductive resources of RI-logic are rather weak, owing to the fact that the inference rules of RI-logic do not include anything corresponding to Leibniz's Law (and owing to the further fact that we have not assumed that identity of person [entails indiscernibility with respect to humanity, divinity or identity of being]).

What van Inwagen leaves implicit (or perhaps obvious) is that the lack of surprise is not simply the absence of Leibniz's Law or the absence of the critical instances of that 'law' (viz., instances governing the theory's key terms 'person', 'humanity', 'divinity'); it's rather that – and this is key – there's simply no *sufficient* condition in the 'RI-logic' governing the key relative-identity predicates. All that is given for the 'definition' of the key family of (relative-identity) predicates are two constraints (corresponding to a syntactic constraint on predicates): namely, that the relative-identity relations are symmetric and transitive.[22] These constraints are *conditional* ones: if you've got the truth of a relative-identity claim then these constraints demand the truth of a few other relative-identity claims. What you don't have is any condition whatsoever that suffices for introducing relative-identity claims into a derivation or theory, except for those that serve as axioms. Since there are many, many (many) symmetric and transitive relations, there

---

[20] For discussion of what such proof achieves (or doesn't) in this context, see Vohánka 2013.

[21] Leibniz's Law in the following passage is either a rule or (detachable) conditional that goes from a true identity claim (say, '$a \sim_N b$' for some identity relation $\sim_N$) to the intersubstitutability of the terms flanking the identity predicate. In short, if '$a \sim_N b$' is true, then anything true of a is true of b too.

[22] Symmetry: *If $a \sim_N b$ then $b \sim_N a$ too.* Transitivity: *If $a \sim_N b$ and $b \sim_N c$ then $a \sim_N c$ too.*

is nothing in 'RI-logic' that demands that the so-called relative-identity relations behave remotely like relative-identity – whatever that behavior might be – unless, of course, all there is to being relative identity is exhausted by symmetry and transitivity together with the rule (which is not explicitly part of the system) that every such relative-identity claim $a \sim_N b$ has as a consequence $Na \wedge Nb$ (i.e., that both a and b satisfy the N predicate).[23] And the absence of a sufficient condition really does make for an unsurprising consistency result.

Let me give an analogy to illuminate the issue, first with brief background on the target case. Having a truth predicate in and for a given language has appeared to be contradictory since ancient times, and certainly the point was made clear by the work of the logician Tarski (1956). The issue is twofold: first, if we have a one-place predicate in the language (such as 'is true'), grammar immediately delivers so-called liar sentences from the predicate and logic's falsity connective (i.e., logical negation): we have sentences like

It's false that Max is true.

The problem arises when, as is perfectly possible, 'Max' denotes the given sentence, that is, when 'Max' denotes 'It is false that Max is true'. And here is the issue: a necessary condition for truth is that it 'release' in the sense that, where $\langle A \rangle$ is a name (e.g., a quotation name, some name like 'Max', or so on), the sentence '$\langle A \rangle$ is true' entails the sentence so named, namely, A itself. (Witness: that 'grass is green' is true entails that grass is green.) But, of course,

---

[23] I use 'a' and 'b' here for singular terms, which are not even in the advanced formal language, except by a backdoor that I do not understand and herein set aside except for the following comment that reflects my confusion: van Inwagen's proposal for using a unique-satisfier predicate 'J' or 'L', which is supposed to have exactly one element of the domain in its extension, does the technical work of denotation; however, if it's available, I do not see how we don't immediately have the resources to define a non-relative identity relation. After all, 'L' is introduced (van Inwagen, 1994, p. 215ff.) as a conjunction of all predicates satisfied by a unique element (viz., Lincoln), and the same for 'J' (viz., Jesus). Presumably, this is available in general for each element of the domain (if it isn't, why is it in this case?). So, let U be schematic for any such unique-satisfier predicate. But, now, define the non-relative identity predicate '$=$' via the schema:

$$x = y \text{ iff } Ux \wedge Uy \text{ for at least some } U.$$

This delivers the result that non-relative identity is a so-called equivalence relation: it's not only symmetric and transitive, but reflexive too (i.e., for every object in the domain, the object stands to itself in the given relation). And reflexivity is at least a sufficient condition for the predicate, a condition resulting from the given definition (together with the substantial resources packed into the idea of unique-satisfier predicates). But the proposed framework is supposed to be neutral on whether there's a non-relative (absolute) equivalence-relation identity relation. But, again, I flag all of this just to set it aside.

the release behavior doesn't differentiate truth from other properties with the given behavior (e.g., 'it's provable that', 'it is known that', or etc.); what is required is a *sufficient* condition too, a rule that tells you what it takes to be true, or tells you, so to speak, that a truth ascription itself is true. In the case of truth, the key sufficient condition is 'capture' behavior, namely, the converse of the release rule: that for any sentence A in the language, A entails the given truth ascription '$\langle A \rangle$ is true'. And with truth thereby well-defined (by not only necessary conditions, but also sufficient), liar sentences cause contradictions, at least if, per the mainstream account of logical consequence, every sentence (including the example Max above) is either true or false (i.e., it's true or its logical negation is true). Quick reflection reveals what Tarski made precise: namely, that liar sentences wind up being true if and only if false, and since, by the mainstream account of logic, they're one or the other, they're both true and false (i.e., they entail a contradiction, which 'explodes' in the mainstream framework).

The foregoing tangent on truth-theoretic (notably, liar) paradox can be forgotten moving forward, but it's useful to illustrate the main reason that relative-identity 'accounts' – at least those with the virtue of metaphysical neutrality – are as yet only promissory: they haven't specified any particular relation of relative identity. To see this, observe that it's relatively simple to prove that, even where logical consequence is per the mainstream (viz., so-called classical logic) account, truth 'can be expressed' in a language, at least if one leaves out any sufficient condition for the target property (i.e., the would-be truth property) – and thereby fails to define the target property in the given theory. More clearly: if you add a one-place predicate 'is true' to the language, and you specify the necessary condition of 'release' but leave out any defining sufficient condition (viz., 'capture') you'll still get liar sentences (because that's just grammar doing its thing); what you won't get is a derivable contradiction.

The question is: have we found a way to avoid the truth-theoretic contradictions by leaving out sufficient conditions that would otherwise define the property? In one sense, yes: we've thereby combined a partially defined property with a bit of (for lack of a better term) 'quietism' or 'agnosticism' about the exact property we're talking about. This can help avoid contradiction, but it's not available to systematic accounts of the target notions.

What would be of great value in turning the promise of relative-identity ideas into well-defined proposals is a so-called 'semantics' for relative-identity relations in christology. At the very least, truth-in-a-model conditions together with falsity-in-a-model conditions for the relations would illuminate the relations, and would fairly immediately deliver sufficient conditions (and necessary conditions) for the notions. As matters stand, at least as far as I can tell, none of this work has been done: there are no accompanying 'true-of' and 'false-of' conditions that define the proposed family of christological predicates.

The promise of a relative-identity strategy towards a consistent (and complete) account of Christ turns on the promise of its key notion: relative identity. Until the full 'logic' (i.e., extra-logical consequence relation) governing the relation is at hand, the promise cannot be sufficiently evaluated. This isn't to say that there is no promise. There is promise; it's just that there are a great many relations that are symmetric and transitive,[24] and until the target key-to-consistency relation (or target family of relations) is specified, the promise remains only promise – interesting promise, but promise.

Let me be clearer: I am not saying that every *strategy* towards a consistent account of Christ must have a detailed, complete theory of the identity relation involved in core christological theses. (A systematic theory requires as much, but a strategy towards such a theory is less demanding.) What I am highlighting is that any strategy that points to the given identity relation – or family of such relations – as the key to avoiding the apparent contradiction(s) of Christ needs to at least fully define the target relation (or even target family of relations) before the strategy can be fruitfully measured against

---

[24] And even many of those relations (i.e., the many symmetric and transitive relations) have simple derivative relations that entail what is not explicitly enforced in 'RI-logic' but is supposed to be an important (so-called meta-theoretic) feature of such relations, namely, that from the truth of '$a \sim_N b$' follows the truth of '$Na \wedge Nb$', and then by logic each conjunct (and so on). But such relations can very obviously diverge widely from what one expects of an identity relation. Example: just off the cuff, here's a cheap route towards such derivative 'relative identity' predicates. Let R be any symmetric and transitive relation that's not reflexive. Now let E be any sortal that can serve grammatically as a predicate. Now define the derivative predicate (open sentence)

$$xR^E y$$

to be

$$xRy \wedge (Ex \wedge Ey)$$

in which case R^E is symmetric, transitive but not reflexive on the given domain, and it also has the necessary but insufficient condition that from the satisfaction of

$$xR^E y$$

follows the satisfaction of

$$Ex \wedge Ey.$$

Observe that R^E has all features that are explicitly noted (although not all enforced) in 'RI-logic'. But there's no reason to think that R^E is a relative-identity relation. (If there is, then the consistency of christological claims in the RI-logic framework is even less surprising than it appears.)

other accounts – accounts that don't point to the identity relation as the key to a consistent christology.

5.7 Epistemic-mystery strategies

Epistemic-mystery strategies, sometimes 'mysterian' strategies,[25] involve a firm twofold commitment to the standard theory of logical consequence (or at least to some 'explosive' theory whereby arbitrary contradictions logically entail all sentences) together with an elaborate epistemological story to the effect that our current epistemic situation cannot but see the apparent contradictions in any viable candidates for the true (and sufficiently complete) christology.[26]

Here, the idea is on one hand straightforward and on the other highly complicated. Much of this strategy, at least in its most developed form,[27] is hand-in-glove with Contradictory Christology as I am advancing it. To begin, the epistemic-mystery strategy maintains that the quest to consistentize Christ is peppered with either heresy (qua departures from the core theory in question) or substantial metaphysical bells and whistles that aren't themselves clearly required by the reality of Christ as revealed in scripture, stamped at Chalcedon, and otherwise uniformly recognized as core christological doctrine. With Contradictory Christology, the epistemic-mystery strategy agrees that the best candidate for a complete account of Christ is an apparently contradictory one. Where the disagreement – and complexity – arises is the next step: the epistemic-mystery account is committed to the standard account of logical consequence or at least some similarly 'explosive'

---

[25] Tuggy (2009, 2011, 2016) uses the term 'mysterian' for such strategies, a term appropriately suggestive of directly related approaches in the philosophy of mind such as the one advocated by McGinn (1991). *Merely terminological note:* Tuggy (2011, p. 209) suggests that he is the source of the neologism 'mysterianism', and also claims (ibid., fn. 6) – truly, to my knowledge – that he is responsible for introducing the term into philosophical theology. Worth flagging is that the term has been around mainstream analytic philosophy for a long time, at least since Owen Flanagan's well-known usage in the philosophy of mind and the clear generalization to other areas of philosophy (Flanagan, 1991, 1992). The particular use of 'mysterian' on either the fundamental problem of christology or the trinity is in exactly the same spirit as the familiar uses in other common areas of philosophy, except for the very explicit tie to the very apparent contradiction at the surface of at least christology.

[26] To use Tuggy's distinction (Tuggy, 2011, 2016) I am focusing on 'positive mysterian' strategies versus those reminiscent of the apophatic or analogical traditions that reject the truth of the core christological claims in the Chalcedon-constrained tradition.

[27] The most developed form is due to Anderson (2007), and this is the implementation that informs my discussion of the strategy.

account (whereby any contradiction logically entails every sentence); hence, on the epistemic-mystery account the apparent contradiction in our best account of Christ is merely apparent. The complexity of the position arises from spelling out an epistemic theory that both accommodates the explicit and rational belief in an apparently contradictory theory with the fact that no contradictory theory is true.

There are sophisticated epistemological theories that serve the epistemic-mystery program.[28] For present purposes, the details of candidate epistemological edifices may be set aside. The central idea of the epistemic-mystery strategy is to accept that the best theory of Christ is apparently contradictory, but to explain the unavoidable apparent contradiction as an unavoidable equivocation the consistent precisification of which – that is, the exact consistent content of which – is beyond our cognitive-cum-epistemic reach. In a nutshell: Christ appears to be contradictory; the appearance is unavoidable in any available candidate for the true and sufficiently complete theory of Christ; but the theory is perfectly acceptable by standard norms because the apparent contradiction, though inevitable (in theories that we can formulate and understand), is only apparently contradictory; the apparent contradiction is due to equivocation the unwrapping of which is beyond our ken. That's the gist.

There is a great deal more that can be said about epistemic-mystery strategies;[29] however, for present purposes, enough has been said to lodge the main elements of my response.

5.7.1 Evaluation: epistemic-mystery accounts

When compared with Contradictory Christology, the epistemic-mystery strategy is inadequate on a number of fronts.

5.7.1.1 Simplicity and epistemic neutrality
In comparison with the contradictory account of Christ advanced in this book, any epistemic-mystery account is bound to be vastly more complicated in general, and significantly less neutral on epistemology or theory of cognition.

---

[28] Anderson (2007) relies on the well-known work of Plantinga (2000).
[29] A useful discussion is by Tuggy (2011, 2016).

There's an old truism that if something looks like a duck, sounds like a duck, behaves like a duck, then, well, it's most probably a duck. One value of the saying is a methodological reminder: the best explanation of an appearance is often that the appearance is veridical. This is especially so when the only reason we're resisting the conclusion that there's truly a duck before us is that our theory of logic leaves no room for ducks (so to speak).

And therein lies the issue of simplicity. On the epistemic-mystery account, we are to abandon the quest for a consistent theory of Christ because the best candidate for a full theory of Christ is inevitably apparently contradictory. (So far so good.) But the simplest explanation of the alleged inevitable appearance of contradiction is that Christ *is* a contradictory being – full stop. Anything less than such a flat-footed explanation of the alleged inevitability of apparent contradiction is to just that extent less simple.

The epistemic-mystery account arrives at the gates of the contradictory Christ but, instead of simply accepting the invitation and stepping through, screeches away with a complex plume of exhaust fueled by background dogma about logical consequence. Free of metaphor: instead of simply accepting that the full truth of Christ is contradictory, epistemic-mystery accounts hold that the apparent truth is inevitably apparently contradictory – but merely apparently so because, as above, the standard account of logical consequence says so. (And the old saying solemnly returns: 'But when I poke it, the being appears to respond as if it really is a duck.' Reply: 'Well, it can't truly be a duck, but it's perfectly good to accept that the being inevitably and in all ways appears to be duck.' In turn: 'But why isn't it a duck?' Reply: 'Because it can't be.')[30]

Beyond simplicity is also the epistemic stake that epistemic-mystery strategies need to put down. Contradictory Christology is neutral with respect to the true epistemology, or at least far closer to neutrality than any epistemic-mystery strategy can sustain. Of course, some epistemological theory is the true theory; however, to stake one's solution to the fundamental 'problem' of christology – to the apparent contradiction of Christ – on a particular candidate or family of candidates strikes me as unduly biased if there's a viable account that avoids said wager.

5.7.1.2 What is the theory?
Another sort of issue concerns the would-be christological theory being advanced (or even defended) along epistemic-mystery lines.

---

[30] To his credit, Anderson (2007) at least gives some arguments against a contradictory approach; however, those arguments have been sufficiently refuted in §4.

What exactly is the theory? On one hand, the underlying theory of logic is one according to which logical consequence is explosive. On the other hand, the would-be complete theory of Christ is supposed to be unavoidably apparently contradictory. But hold on! If the theory appears, for all we can see, contradictory and is also closed under classical logic, the theory is trivial: it contains all sentences of the language of the theory, including not only each and every heretical sentence (e.g., 'Christ is a concert of two distinct persons', etc.) but also flat-out theological absurdities (e.g., 'Christ is Satan' or 'God is pure evil' or etc.). So perhaps the target theory is not closed under logic? In this case, why think that it's contradictory? The claims 'Christ is divine' and 'Christ is human' jointly entail the apparent contradiction of Christ (e.g., the derivation on page 120); however, if we refuse to close our theory under logic or some theological-specific consequence relation, we can easily avoid the contradictory consequences – just walk away, and let the 'theory' of Christ be a grab bag of claims sans their otherwise explosive consequences. Presumably, then, abandoning the idea that theology, as with other truth-seeking disciplines, aims to provide a complete theory closed under logic is not the aim of the epistemic-mystery strategy. (If it were, one could drop the elaborate epistemological theory and concomitant cognitive theory and just avoid the entailments of one's core claims.) The trouble is that it remains unclear what the would-be theory of Christ is supposed to be on an epistemic-mystery account. And this raises another unclarity: if it's unclear what the theory of Christ is supposed to be (aside from being inevitably apparently contradictory), why think that 'the theory' – that is, the target christology or, generally, theology – is apparently contradictory? I do not know the answer, but the question points to a related problem with epistemic-mystery strategies vis-à-vis the advanced contradictory account (see §5.7.1.3.).

5.7.1.3 An alternative account: gappy christology
There seems to be a closely related strategy that avoids the epistemological edifice while achieving the other desiderata of epistemic-mystery strategies. My aim is to say just enough to illustrate an option that appears to deliver key desiderata of the epistemic-mystery account without the need for epistemic mystery or sophisticated epistemological commitments. Here, instead of the glut-theoretic account one pursues a gap-theoretic account while rejecting the standard norm governing 'proper acceptance' or 'proper assertion' or the like:[31]

---

[31] For precedent see Beall and Ripley 2004, and also Maudlin 2004.

- Firmly reject that some contradictions are true (i.e., that there are gluts).
- Reject that only true claims are properly assertible or properly acceptable: some gaps are properly assertible.
- The true theory of Christ is invariably gappy with respect to the full description of Christ, a description that involves gappy claims – claims that are neither true nor false.
- One mystery of 'the full account' of Christ is that if true then it's an incomplete description, and if it's a complete description then it's untrue (because contains some gappy claims).[32]
- Distinguish between 'accurate description' of Christ and 'true claim about Christ'. (This is tightly wound with the points above.)

On this sort of account, the best theory of Christ – if 'full' or 'complete description' – does indeed appear to be contradictory, just as the epistemic-mystery strategy claims. Moreover, per a key desideratum of the epistemic-mystery strategy, absolutely no contradictions are true (perhaps, depending on exact details, not even logically possibly true). But instead of appealing to an elaborate epistemological edifice to explain the apparent contradiction of Christ, one instead points to a rejection of the standard norm of assertible descriptions of an object; in turn, one rejects that the full description of Christ involves only truths. The full description of Christ involves no falsehoods, on this account; it's just that it involves some gaps, which are untrue.

This sort of story, subject to details (none of which are herein supplied), strikes me as delivering a better non-contradictory account of the apparent contradiction of Christ than the epistemic-mystery strategy can otherwise provide. Here, the appearance of contradiction is tied directly to the untrue-but-gappy description of Christ involved in the 'full description' of God incarnate, a description that involves negation-inconsistent claims: *it's true that Christ is immutable* but *it's false that Christ is immutable*, and so on. Again, on the proposed account, such claims are neither false nor, alas, true; they are simply required by any full description of the strangeness of Christ's being.

As far as I can see, provided that the details can be sufficiently drawn out, such a gap-theoretic christology is more promising than accounts

---

[32] The exact details will be telling: if logic is classical then the 'full' theory will explode into a mess of gappy claims on top of the proper subset of true claims; if the logic is (say) FDE, as I have advanced it, then the 'full' theory needn't explode into the trivial theory; it will nonetheless be untrue (because containing gaps).

that demand the inevitable appearance of contradictions but tie the inevitability (and rational endorsement) of such apparent contradictions to a sophisticated epistemological theory. A simpler account is that the appearance of such contradictions is explained by their necessity in the full description of Christ, a description that upends the tables of the standard norm of assertible descriptions (because upends the norm according to which only true descriptions are properly assertible).

Still, even if, as I think, such a gap-theoretic account is more promising than the epistemic-mystery route, it ultimately fares no better than the epistemic-mystery route when compared with the simplicity of the corresponding contradictory account. After all, why not just have both the complete and true theory – contradictory as it is? The response ultimately points to the dogma against gluts: we should reject that contradictions can be true, ergo should reject that any contradictions are true of Christ. My reply, as this book lays out, is this: why is that? Pending a good explanation, the proposed distinction between *accurate* and *true* descriptions of Christ remains under-motivated.

5.8 Contradictory precedents?

At least one theologian (viz., J. V. Dahms) has claimed that various standard ideas about logic should be rejected in order to accommodate the apparent contradictions in christian theology. Dahms (1978) thereby deserves credit for pointing in the direction of accepting a better account of logic than the standard one; however, Dahms' positive view is not clearly a forerunner to the account advanced in this book. In particular, Dahms' view appears to be that the true theology is simply free from the constraints of logic, that logic itself is not in fact universal – that some true theories are true only by going against the demands of logic.[33]

None of this 'freedom from logic' is involved in the view I advance. True theories – be they in physics, mathematics, philosophy, theology, or any realm – are one and all constrained by logic (i.e., by logical consequence, by logical entailment). True theories, if they're to be systematic and complete with respect to their target phenomenon, are bound by logic. Logic, contrary

---

[33] Fideists, at least as understood per Plantinga (1983), also reject the universal reach of logic on true theories, at least if they take theology to be a true theory. And Martin Luther might have likewise rejected the universal reach of logic on true theories (Lehmann, 1971, p. 256).

to the picture suggested by Dahms, is universal, applying to all true theories if any. The question is whether the correct account of logic is one wherein logic recognizes the possibility of 'true contradictions'. Dahms' picture is one in which the answer is negative; my account, per previous chapters, is one in which the answer is affirmative.

Beyond Dahms, no theologian or theologically inclined philosopher has advocated a specific contradictory theology, at least not a systematic, logic-bound theology, let alone a specific contradictory christology. There simply is no precedent for a systematic but logically contradictory (i.e., 'glutty') christian theology, where being systematic (in this context) involves, among other things, being explicit and precise about both the source of the target gluts – the true contradictions – and the relation of entailment (consequence) governing the systematic theory (theology, christology, etc.) in question.[34]

None of this is to say that theologians over the centuries haven't witnessed the apparent contradiction of Christ. Clearly, many – many many many – sincere, competent, and devoted thinkers have witnessed the remarkable contradiction, with such witness reflected in otherwise puzzling passages from Tertullian, Leo (the Tome), Luther, Ratzinger, Barth, a host of mystics and, perhaps especially, fideists and some so-called existentialists (e.g., Kierkegaard) who, in recognition of the contradictory Christ, erroneously declare that the truth breaks the bounds of logic. But seeing the contradiction and explicitly affirming it in a systematic theology are different. The usual response by those who have explicitly remarked on the contradiction of Christ is that the contradiction breaks the bounds of logic – the true theology is beyond logic's reach. Not so. Not at all. As I have tried to make plain in this book, the truth is within the bounds of logic; the truth rather powerfully shows how far the bounds reach when transcendence and immanence unite in a human-divine baby in a manger.

---

[34] Cotnoir (2018b) deserves credit for advocating the exploration of systematic, glut-theoretic christian theologies in general. Cotnoir's given work is an initial, partial exploration of different glut-theoretic options and some of their issues. I'm in agreement with Cotnoir's main methodological point that such work has been neglected to the detriment of systematic, truth-seeking theology; however, unlike the salient issues in Cotnoir's given paper, the incarnation of God, on my view, is the key motivation, a being who appears to be contradictory by exemplifying contrary natures. (But see §6 for my first steps towards a contradictory account of the trinity in relation to the contradictory truth of Christ.)

In addition to Dahms, others who may've been working towards a precise, logically bound christian theology are Hegel and Florensky, as discussed, respectively, by Ficara (2009) and Rojek (2019). I remain unclear on any substantial similarities between their projects and my own. I leave this to future debate.

6
Towards the trinity

*The Trinity, one God, of whom are all things, through whom are all
things, in whom are all things. Thus the Father and the Son and the
Holy Spirit, and each of these by Himself, is God, and at the same
time they are all one God; and each of them by Himself is a complete
substance, and yet they are all one substance. The Father is not the
Son nor the Holy Spirit; the Son is not the Father nor the Holy Spirit;
the Holy Spirit is not the Father nor the Son: but the Father is only
Father, the Son is only Son, and the Holy Spirit is only Holy Spirit.*

– Augustine, *On Christian Doctrine*

6.1 Important disclaimer

The trinity is often thought to be one of the central sources of contradiction
in christian theology, certainly by those who charge that christian theology's
two distinctive doctrines (viz., incarnation and trinity) are contradictory.
§§1–5 argue that the truth of the incarnation is contradictory, that Christ
himself is a contradictory being. Given the contradiction of Christ's very
being, it's very natural to think that the trinity is also contradictory, inher-
iting (so to speak) contradictions from the contradictory Christ who is
essentially God – the one and only god, who is three persons, one of whom is
Christ. But is the trinity contradictory? Are the contradictions of the trinity
(if any) simply consequences of Christ's contradictory being? Are there
contradictions that are both true of the trinity and independent from the
contradictions of Christ? These are questions on which this chapter touches
but – and this is a very important qualification – just barely touches.

There are many critical issues that anything more than a sketch needs to
address. Some issues are hermeneutical or interpretive, including accounts
of how 'is God' and 'is consubstantial with God [the Father]' are related in

The Contradictory Christ. Jc Beall, Oxford University Press (2021). © Jc Beall.
DOI: 10.1093/oso/9780198852360.003.0006

historical works of orthodox trinitarian theory (Anatolios, 2011; Ayres, 2004; Barnes, 1998; Coakley, 1999, 2004; Wolfson, 1964). Other issues involve fundamental methodological principles, including – but by no way limited to – issues reflected in the 'divide' between so-called Western and Eastern methodological approaches (Ayres, 2004; Barnes, 1998; Coakley, 1999; Cross, 2002*b*). Other issues are theoretically fundamental in the sense that each trinitarian theory must supply answers – indeed, perhaps 'axioms' – such as whether, as I assume throughout this chapter, trinitarian identity is in fact a binary relation, and if so whether it's an 'absolute' or 'relative' relation or even something in between (Brower and Rea, 2005; Coakley, 2013; Martinich, 1978, 1979; McCall, 2010; McCall and Rea, 2009; Rea, 2003, 2011). And, of course, lest the trinitarian theory be untethered from orthodox or standard tradition, any account of the trinity must navigate the trio of persistent trinitarian heresies (viz., subordination, modalism, polytheism), heresies that often arise, as in christology, from a quest to avoid apparent contradictions in the trinity (Anatolios, 2011; Crisp and Sanders, 2014; Holmes, 2012; McCall and Rea, 2009).

The disclaimer for this chapter is just this: the current chapter deals with only one issue in the vast number of issues concerning the trinity, and does so in at most an exploratory fashion, and at best a first-little-steps manner.

The aim of this chapter is simply to answer a question that arises in the face of Christ's contradictory being: namely, what, then, of any apparent contradictions in the trinity? Are such appearances also veridical? And even on this question the current discussion is highly limited in its reach. This chapter looks not to debates about conciliar-text interpretations or the would-be history of terminology and philosophical terms surrounding the councils and creeds that affirm the trinity; the chapter instead simply takes the contradictions of Christ as read, and in turn explores one way in which truths about the trinity – and, specifically (and only), truths involving the would-be (non-relative) trinitarian-identity relation (more on which below) – might naturally be contradictory, even independent from the contradictions of Christ. While it seems to me that any systematic account of the trinity must define the relation of trinitarian identity (involved in claims such as 'God is the Son' and 'the Son is not the Father' and 'the Father is God', etc.), no such account is a full account of the trinity itself. The aim here is only to give a very simple and natural thumbnail sketch of how contradictions may naturally arise in the trinity. The sketch is just that: a mere sketch.

The preceding chapters have advanced and defended an account accord-ing to which Christ is a contradictory being. My aim in this chapter is to sketch the most obvious direction for a unified account of both the incarnation and trinity, one in which, focusing only on the predicates that are either true of God or false of God, both Christ and the trinity are contradictory in different but natural ways, the contradictions of Christ, per the preceding chapters, arising from his extraordinary 2-natured being, the contradictions of the trinity from the extraordinary relation of *identity*-with-difference and *difference*-with-identity.

The aim of this chapter – to belabor the disclaimer once more – is not to resolve the issue once and for all. My own thinking is insufficiently settled to say, as this book says of Christ, that the right account of the trinity is contradictory. I remain very open to the possibility of a contradictory trinity; however, the actuality requires a great deal more reflection – too much more for this chapter. This chapter simply charts the most obvious path.

Before turning directly to the trinity and the key trinitarian-identity claims, I review a few methodological rules of thumb, mainly for the sake of keeping the larger background picture in mind.

6.2 Some methodological rules of thumb

Logic recognizes both gluts and gaps. This doesn't mean that the full truth of the world is either glutty or gappy; logic recognizes pigs that fly faster than the speed of light, but this doesn't mean that the truth of our world involves flying pigs.

How do we decide when to recognize gluts or gaps – or even other 'classical' but still far-out logical possibilities as actualities? I don't know. And I don't think that anybody knows. In the end, what we do is the best we can with rough rules of thumb combined with hard work and sincere inquiry.

6.2.1 Go simple and natural

As a very important rule of thumb, I follow a flat-footed dictum: go for the simplest, most natural explanation of the apparent phenomenon.

This dictum is not only imprecise; its key notions are highly sensitive to other theories that we hold fixed at the time of inquiry. For example, were we to erroneously hold to the mainstream account of logical consequence, no glut-theoretic explanation of any phenomenon would appear to be either simple or natural; it'd be absurd – logically so, and so absurd full stop.

The terms 'simple' and 'natural', in the given context, are not only highly sensitive to other theories we hold; they may be near-impossible to adequately define for all cases whatsoever. But for all that, the principle still serves as a useful rule of thumb. The dictum, despite its imprecision, is a methodological principle that guides us – certainly guides me in my pursuit of truth.

6.2.2 Go for a complete story

Another rule of thumb: go for the full truth – deciding, for each sentence in the language of the theory, whether it's true or false.

This principle is a sort of methodological-completeness principle that has the effect of pushing away from gaps (i.e., gappy sentences). The aim is for the full truth to validate at least one of $\dagger A$ and $\neg A$, for each sentence A in the language. Logic itself doesn't force this; however, our pursuit of complete theories does.

Of course, like any of these principles, this one can be overturned in the face of 'recalcitrant data' that persists in appearing to be gappy. (One might think that cases of so-called vagueness serve as just such recalcitrant data about certain phenomena. Example: for what number n is it true that at exactly n seconds old you became an adult?) Still, our pursuit of the truth is guided by aiming at the full truth, free of gaps.

6.2.3 Go for a consistent story

Another rule of thumb: go for a consistent theory – deciding, for each sentence in the language of the theory, whether it's just-true or just-false.

This principle is a sort of methodological-consistency principle that has the effect of pushing away from gluts (i.e., glutty sentences). The aim is for the full truth to validate at most one of $\dagger A$ and $\neg A$, for each sentence A in the language. Logic itself doesn't force this; however, our pursuit of consistent theories does.

6.2.4 Putting it all together

Needless to say, there are abnormal phenomena that give pause: the familiar principles above, despite their imprecision, push in different directions with no further guidance on which hay bale to eat (so to speak). But we still eat hay. We still find our way.

In the case of Christ, the persistent appearance of contradiction – as witnessed by the longstanding fundamental 'problem' – is simply and naturally explained by Christ's being a contradictory being. Of course, this explanation goes against the consistency principle (§6.2.3) while walking the line of completeness (§6.2.2), at least with respect to the given properties. But in the incarnation case, the option of bucking completeness in favor of consistency via gaps is a clearly defective course: rejecting that Christ has the standard properties (e.g., mutability and immutability, etc.) is a logical option; however, it steps decidedly away from the reality that we thought we were describing (at least when describing a *fully divine* and *fully human* reality).[1] For this reason, the gappy approach – which walks the consistent line while bucking the completeness line – appears to be more complicated or less natural than the glutty one, which bucks the consistency line but walks the completeness line.

And so goes my simple thinking: Christ appears to be contradictory; the simplest and most natural explanation of the appearance is that Christ is a contradictory being. This account is in line with the goal of 'full truth' at the expense of consistency. But for all that I can tell, the expense is no cost; it's just the way of a unique, radical, and extraordinary aspect of reality – the incarnation of God, the full-on unity of transcendence and immanence in exactly one person, a human who is God. This is foolishness to the consistency norm, but simple, true, and complete for all that.

The broader question at hand is at least twofold: namely, whether there are apparent contradictions of God that are independent of the contradictions of Christ, and if so whether such apparent contradictions are simply and naturally explained along non-glut-theoretic lines, for example via *gaps* – claims of God that are neither true of nor false of God – or even some simple and natural 'classical' (i.e., gap-free and glut-free) explanation.

My disappointing answer in this chapter: I don't know. What I do know is that there's no logical bar against treating any other would-be theological contradictions as gaps (or even, possibly, along 'classical' lines). But logical

---

[1] One might, as the upstream meaning-change accounts sometimes do (see §5.5.1), resist rejecting the given *pairs* of properties – which demands gaps, as far as I can see – and hoe a complete (and gap-free) account by treating exactly one member of each pair as true of (false of) Christ. This, from my perspective, appears to be imbalanced in ways that are at least avoided by a gappy account. In any event, even by the upstream theorists' lights, such a route involves a meaning change away from what we thought we were talking about.

bars, as per §2, are few and far between. The issue in this chapter is whether commonly cited trinity-driven contradictions are best treated as gluts of God, even if such would-be gluts don't trace directly to Christ, the source, as I've said in previous chapters, of gluts in the world. The issue deserves its own book-length discussion.[2] For present purposes, my aim in what follows is simply to sketch the most obvious natural route towards a unified contradictory account of both the incarnation and trinity. The contradiction of Christ, for purposes of this chapter, I treat as read. The contradictions of the trinity are the remaining focus.

6.3 Accounting for the trinity

Two doctrines distinguish christian theology from its traditional monotheistic cousins: the incarnation and the trinity. The former, as I've discussed throughout the book, is simply and naturally understood along contradictory lines: the full truth of the incarnation (ergo, the full truth of God) involves gluts. The question concerns the latter doctrine – the trinity. And here one naturally expects that if one person, who is God, is contradictory, God is contradictory. And that, of course, is correct: God is contradictory, at least in virtue of Christ's contradictory being. The question is whether there are further contradictions true of God that are not directly traced back, so to speak, to Christ. I remain open on the answer, but in what follows I assume, as only a tentative assumption, an affirmative answer based on what I take to be a natural thought: namely, that any apparent contradictions arising from God's triune nature are best explained via similarities and differences among the three persons each of whom is the one and only God.

Accounts of the trinity can exceed not only a few pages (to put matters mildly); they can differ widely in what they're trying to explain, and how they're trying to explain it. The full slate of such issues is beyond this chapter. For present purposes, I focus on three basic tasks for any account of the trinity.

- *Trinitarian identity.* Specify the target identity relation involved in the core trinitarian theses. (This involves, at the very least, specifying

---

[2] I am working towards just such a discussion, and this chapter serves as a small pointer to only some of the issues involved in the future work.

necessary and sufficient conditions for the relation to hold, and specifying any notable features of the relation so defined.)

- *Counting by trinitarian identity.* Specify the *counting conventions* associated with the trinitarian-identity relation. (This involves, at the very least, specifying the target senses of 'there is one God' and 'there are three persons each of whom is God'.)
- *Explanation.* Specify an explanation that motivates the given account. (This involves, at the very least, specifying how properties of the three persons and properties of the one and only God explain the status of target trinitarian-identity claims.)

Saying just this much, even if said well, is to say too little. But for present purposes, the little bit said suffices to highlight key issues on the topic of would-be trinitarian contradiction.

6.4   Whereof trinity-driven contradictions?

Let me begin by repeating, per §2, that logic itself (i.e., logical vocabulary), on my view, is predicate-free: there are no predicates in the logical vocabulary, and hence there is no identity predicate in the logical vocabulary. Identity is not topic-neutral enough to be involved in all true and full-as-possible theories. Accordingly, it's the job of the theorist (including theological theorist, including any would-be systematic theologian) to specify the identity relation(s) involved in one's would-be true theory. When it comes to (at least target) candidates for the true theory of the trinity, it is fairly obvious that the identity relation is not the typical one often called 'classical first-order identity'. After all, that relation is not only an equivalence relation;[3] it also validates intersubstitutability of 'identicals', that is: if some predicate P is true of object x, and if x is identical to an object y, then predicate P is true of y too.[4] But clearly such features are not involved in the trinitarian-identity theses:

---

[3] A binary (i.e., 2-place) relation R on a domain D of objects is said to be an *equivalence relation* iff it's reflexive, symmetric, and transitive on D. In that order: R is *reflexive* (on D) iff every element of D stands in R to itself; the relation is *symmetric* (on D) iff for any objects x and y in D, if x stands in R to y then y stands in R to x; and the relation is *transitive* (on D) iff for any objects x, y and z in D, if x stands in R to y, and y stands in R to z, then x stands in R to z too.

[4] Strictly speaking, by 'predicate' here I mean what logicians mean by 'open sentence', which is basically any sentence where you remove at least one singular term (i.e., a term that picks out an individual, a term like a name, a denoting definite description, etc.).

So the Father is God; the Son is God; and the Holy Ghost is God. And yet they are not three Gods; but one God. – *Athanasian Creed*.

The oddness of the trinity is its identity-with-difference or difference-with-identity:

1. One:
    (a) The Father is identical to God.
    (b) The Son is identical to God.
    (c) The Spirit is identical to God.

2. Three:
    (a) The Father is not identical to the Son.
    (b) The Son is not identical to the Spirit.
    (c) The Spirit is not identical to the Father.

It's very obviously the case that, unless the theory (i.e., the theology) is the trivial theology (and it's not), the trinitarian-identity relation is not the so-called classical (first-order) identity relation; for intersubstitutability of identicals is enough to 'trivialize' the entire theory – quickly entailing that every object is identical and not identical to every other object, and thereby every predicate is both true and false of every object. This is the paradigm of absurdity, and is obviously not what's going on in the trinitarian-identity theory. Moreover, intersubstitutability of identicals aside, even transitivity of the relation is fairly obviously (though not necessarily) absent in the given theses' identity relation. After all, without hidden complications elsewhere, transitivity would collapse the minimal distinctions in the given Godhead: were transitivity in play, (1) would entail that each of the subjects is identical to the others, and this trivializes the claims in (2), at least in the standard account of logic in which classical first-order identity is often cited.[5]

Some might, as some have (Anderson, 2007), argue that the given appearance of trinitarian-driven contradiction is as clear as the fundamental contradictions of Christ's two-natured being. I'm not among those who say as much. From my perspective, that the target identity relation is non-transitive – and certainly does not validate intersubstitutability of identicals – is so plain, so naturally suggested by the target theses, that to assume (for what reason?) that the relation is otherwise (let alone that it's the classical first-order identity relation) strikes me as in very plain need of motivation.

---

[5] For an elementary walk through some of these issues, see Martinich 1978.

To be sure, if one (erroneously) thought that logic itself comes equipped with an identity predicate then that predicate is in the vocabulary of theology as much as any other bit of logical vocabulary is in the language. But even in that case, why think that the would-be logical identity predicate is the relation involved in the trinitarian-identity theses? And even if there's some good reason to think as much, there's a follow-up question: why think that the logical predicate behaves per the classical account of logic? For all that I can see, there simply aren't good reasons to think that the trinitarian-identity relation is transitive (let alone validates intersubstitutability of identicals). Indeed, the appearance is clearly the opposite: it looks, from the get-go, to be at least non-transitive.[6]

Where, then, are the apparent contradictions of the trinity? If there are any, the contradictions help to explain *why* trinitarian identity is not transitive. This, at least tentatively, is the central idea I sketch here: the would-be contradictions arising from the trinity explain the failure of transitivity (and of substitutability); they aren't in any way a result of the validity of such properties.

6.5 Trinitarian identity

What, then, is the target non-transitive identity relation (that invalidates intersubstitutability too)? There are many (many) candidates; however, in the present context, where, as per §2, I hold that logical consequence is per the FDE account of consequence, the most obvious first step is to look for the relation in the vicinity of FDE resources. Of course, as above, logic itself does not have an identity predicate in its (topic-neutral, universal) vocabulary. Still, there are natural routes towards identity relations that make at least partial use of the logical vocabulary, and in particular of logic's material conditional.[7]

---

[6] Note that it's in the face of such a clear appearance that so-called relative-identity strategies hit the ground running: they try to explain the apparent abnormality of the trinitarian-identity relation via would-be relative-identity relations whereby we don't have *being identical* simpliciter; we have only *identical-sub-god, identical-sub-person*, etc. These ideas have a lot going for them, and might ultimately be right, but as yet I remain unconvinced that the trinity demands relative-identity relations (however ultimately they are defined). But I leave this for future discussion.

[7] See §2 for a review of the logical vocabulary and the behavior of logic's (material) conditional.

The idea behind what some philosophers call 'absolute identity' is a so-called second-order idea:[8] the identity of objects x and y amounts to the (second-order) claim that for any property P whatsoever, P is true (respectively, false) of x *if and only if (iff)* P is true (respectively, false) of y.[9] In effect, one can think of this idea in terms of 'conditions' (technically, open sentences) specified by the given predicates (strictly, open sentences):

- That x and y are identical entails – and, conversely, is entailed by – the truth of the biconditional: P is true (respectively, false) of x *iff* P is true (respectively, false) of y, for *all predicates/conditions P*.

In effect, then, one just goes through the target predicates and considers, where 'a' and 'b' are names of two objects, all sentences of the form

$$Pa \text{ iff } Pb$$

(even though, note, the P in question can be any open sentence into whose 'open slots' the given names are plugged). If all such biconditionals are at least true, then the target identity statement between a and b is likewise at least true. Likewise, mutatis mutandis, for falsity.

For example, if there's a predicate that's just-true of x but just-false of y, then x and y fail to be identical. Moreover, since some predicates can be both true of and false of an object (i.e., glutty with respect to the object), x and y can be identical in virtue of all predicates being true of both objects, even if some predicates are also false of one of them.[10] There are many (many) other available identity relations available in an FDE-based setting, but this one is the most obvious, and is in keeping with the idea that if P is glutty with respect to an object, it's still true of the object, and no less so, for whatever such degree-theoretic language is worth, than P's being just-true of an object. This is the view of glutty predicates that I endorse, and the one that figures in my account of Christ throughout this book.

---

[8] The distinction between *first-order* versus *second-order* claims is precisely specified in theories of so-called second-order consequence (and third-order consequence and so on), but the details can be set aside here. For a fairly user-friendly introduction to such ideas (though in the context of a particular epistemic program in the philosophy of mathematics) see Shapiro 1991.

[9] Such so-called higher-order quantification, on my view, is beyond logic; however, it's perfectly common in the languages of many true theories.

[10] Again, reflection on the material conditional as discussed in §2 reinforces these ideas.

What's important to observe is that the foregoing approach to so-called absolute identity is not just familiar and common (e.g., it's the one behind the familiar classical first-order identity relation); it's also an account whose details turn on the details of the biconditional involved – the 'iff' on the right-hand side – and the account of logical consequence in the background. Logic here, as throughout, is FDE (see §2). But while logic has a conditional – the relatively weak material conditional – one can certainly use theory-specific conditionals for the target biconditional, conditionals that go beyond the resources of logical vocabulary but are available as extra-logical resources. That's an option, but I keep things simple and stick with the weaker (logical) conditional.

I take the target biconditional – the biconditional involved in the defining 'schema' of trinitarian identity – to be nothing more nor less than logic's own material (bi-) conditional, defined per usual out of logic's conditional and logic's conjunction connective.[11] In particular, then, where $\leftrightarrow$ is the FDE biconditional and, for clarity, '$\simeq$' is the target trinitarian-identity predicate, '$\mathcal{P}$' is a stand-in for all target predicates, and 'a' and 'b' stand-in for names, the approach under discussion is just as above:

- *Trinitarian-identity relation.* That $a \simeq b$ is true (respectively, false) entails – and, conversely, is entailed by – the truth (respectively, falsity) of *all* instances of $\mathcal{P}a \leftrightarrow \mathcal{P}b$, for each individual predicate $\mathcal{P}$ in the language of the theory.

In other words, to find out whether the claim $a \simeq b$ is true, you look to all given biconditionals $Pa \leftrightarrow Pb$ involving all relevant predicates P. The way to think of this account of the trinitarian-identity relation, at least for present purposes, is as a 'schema' over all target biconditionals,[12] and the entire schema is in effect like a conjunction – a conjunction of all the individual biconditionals involving each different predicate in the target set of predicates. A key fact concerns trinitarian-identity claims that are just-false: namely, a given identity claim

$$a \simeq b$$

---

[11] The definition, per §2, is this: the material conditional $A \rightarrow B$ is defined, as is usual in logic, as $\neg A \lor B$, the disjunction of the negated 'antecedent' and the 'consequent'. In turn, the material biconditional $\leftrightarrow$ is defined via conjunction of two such conditionals: $A \leftrightarrow B$ is defined to be $(A \rightarrow B) \land (B \rightarrow A)$.

[12] Alternatively, the so-called schema here can also just be a second-order universal generalization over all target predicates and names.

is just-false (i.e., not even at least true)[13] if and only if there's at least one instance of the defining schema (i.e., one particular biconditional)

$$Pa \leftrightarrow Pb$$

which is just-false. Accordingly, so long as there's at least one predicate P (e.g., 'begotten', 'crucified', 'proceeds-via-Son') which is just-true of one object but just-false of another, the trinitarian-identity predicate '$\simeq$' is just-false of the given pair of objects. In other words, if

$$Pa$$

is just-true (just-false) and

$$Pb$$

is just-false (just-true) then the biconditional $Pa \leftrightarrow Pb$ is just-false, and so, by definition, $a \simeq b$ is just-false too. That's the basic idea. And as per §6.5, the given 'schema' (strictly, the universally quantified second-order biconditional) is at least true so long as there's no instance which is not at least true.

This is the first-cab-off-the-block approach to (non-relative) identity, and I shall focus on this approach here. Again, this is the standard approach when one pursues a non-relative identity relation, whether it's in the mainstream-logic setting or other settings. One might, in turn, fiddle with the target biconditional so as to get different properties for the target relation; however, as above, I simply follow the first-thought course of using logic's own – however weak – material (bi-) conditional, letting the properties of trinitarian identity fall out in turn.

6.5.1 Properties of trinitarian identity

Whatever else the trinitarian-identity relation may be, it is pretty clearly not, as above, an equivalence relation (i.e., reflexive, symmetric and transitive)

---

[13] I am setting aside the possibility of gaps for present purposes.

that validates intersubstitutability of identicals. And my current proposal fits the bill, at least on bucking some of these properties.[14]

6.5.1.1 On reflexivity of trinitarian identity

One immediate upshot of the proposed account is that, unless the logical possibility of gaps is removed as a theoretical (indeed, theological) impossibility with respect to God (the Father, Son and Spirit), the reflexivity of identity statements is invalid (according to the target theological consequence relation):[15] if P is gappy with respect to God (notation, '$\mathfrak{g}$' for God), then the biconditional

$$P\mathfrak{g} \leftrightarrow P\mathfrak{g}$$

is equally gappy, and hence not even at least true, and hence the corresponding trinitarian-identity claim

$$\mathfrak{g} \cong \mathfrak{g}$$

is likewise gappy – and hence neither true nor false.

This consequence does not strike me as problematic in the face of the logical (or, indeed, even theological) possibility of gaps; however, if it were a problem – especially a theological problem – then the possibility of gaps for God can be removed, treated in turn as a theological impossibility, something logically possible but, for purposes of the true theory, theoretically impossible (showing up in no acceptable models of the theory).

While I remain open to the option of some gaps for God, my principal aim in this chapter is to sketch the most obvious route towards a unified account of contradictions in the incarnation and trinity. Accordingly, for purposes of core trinitarian-identity theses, we can restrict (higher-order) quantification (over properties in the definition of trinitarian identity) to those and only those predicates that are either true or false of God (and so true or false of the Father, Son, and Spirit). Restricting to this set of

---

[14] Martin Pleitz kindly sent his 'Münster One Workshop' slides (2015), which he presented at a metaphysics workshop. (I was not at said workshop.) The slides show that Pleitz and I are in agreement, at least in effect, with this first-step approach to non-relative trinitarian identity, although Pleitz's account, very much unlike mine, is driven by a particular metaphysical account of 'unity' the details of which I haven't explored (Priest, 2014). I should note that while his metaphysical pursuit leads to the same basic first-step approach, Pleitz's work seems to be disconnected from what I take to be the critical contradictions arising from Christ's 2-natured being. (This isn't at all a criticism; it's an observation.) I should also note, just to be very clear, that I make no claims whatsoever about the metaphysics of the trinity here.

[15] Recall, from §2, that $A \rightarrow A$ is not logically valid according to FDE; hence, nor is the corresponding biconditional.

predicates delivers reflexivity of trinitarian identity, and for present purposes I focus only on the restricted set of predicates. The target issues of trinitarian-identity contradictions – and especially gluts of God whose source is the trinity, and not simply the contradictions of Christ – are evident even on this restricted focus.[16]

6.5.1.2 On symmetry of trinitarian identity

Given that symmetry of logic's biconditional is logically valid, the symmetry of trinitarian identity is thereby logic-backed. The reason that $\leftrightarrow$ is symmetric in FDE is that the 'logical form' of such $\leftrightarrow$ statements is conjunction – namely, $A \wedge B$, where A and B are conditionals (viz., logic's material conditional) – and logical conjunction 'commutes' in the sense that $A \wedge B$ and $B \wedge A$ are logically equivalent (each logically entails the other), for any A and B whatsoever.

6.5.1.3 On (non-) transitivity of trinitarian identity

There's a very clear and natural explanation for why the transitivity of trinitarian identity is *in*valid, with or without the possibility of gaps (a possibility that, only for purposes of this chapter, I'm setting aside for simplicity): namely, that the possibility of gluts invalidates transitivity, not only logically invalidates it, in the sense that, where $\vdash$ is logical consequence,

$$A \leftrightarrow B, B \leftrightarrow C \nvdash A \leftrightarrow C$$

but invalidates it according to the true account of the trinity (which, for present purposes, we're taking to demand such gluts). Where $\vdash_\Theta$ is the target theological consequence relation:

$$A \leftrightarrow B, B \leftrightarrow C \nvdash_\Theta A \leftrightarrow C$$

To see this, let A be just-true; let B be a glut (both true and false); let C be just-false. Now, the FDE material biconditional, like any material biconditional, is at least true so long as both sentences flanking the biconditional are both at least true or both at least false: as standardly put, the truth of the

---

[16] Indeed, for simplicity, I focus on just a few predicates to illuminate the target issues, namely, 'divine', 'human', 'person', 'peccable', 'sinless', and both 'begotten' and 'proceeding via Son' – the last one, if overly controversial, can be replaced with any predicate that is definitive of the Spirit, for example, 'Comforter' or 'Advocate' or 'Counselor' (or the like) per John 16:17.

bicoditional ensures that the pair of claims are either true together or false together, and that's that.[17] In the given possibility in which A is just-true, B is glutty (true and false), and C is just-false, the glut – being, in the case at hand, a special case of intimately unified contrary properties – is the link that breaks transitivity: $A \leftrightarrow B$ is at least true because the given claims (viz., A and B) are both at least true together, and $B \leftrightarrow C$ is at least true because the given claims are both at least false together. Hence, in the given case we have

- At least true: $A \leftrightarrow B$
- At least true: $B \leftrightarrow C$

but, because the pair of elements A and C are neither at least true together nor at least false together, we have

- Just-false: $A \leftrightarrow C$

And so there are at least relevant possibilities that invalidate – serve as counterexample to the validity of the – transitivity of $\leftrightarrow$. Of course, logical possibilities can be – and often are, and often must be – ruled out by true theories; however, the true theology, as I have argued, has gluts at its very core, and some such logical possibilities remain theoretical (in this case, theological) possibilities. Accordingly, transitivity of $\leftrightarrow$ in the true theology, or at least the fragment concerning the trinity, is invalid for reasons above.

With the non-transitivity of $\leftrightarrow$, which defines the proposed relation of trinitarian identity, we also get the non-transitivity of $\simeq$ as a natural effect. (The truth of such identity claims turns, by definition, on the truth of the corresponding biconditionals. Given that the biconditionals are not transitive, the defined relation is not transitive either.) This is a positive feature of the relation in the given context.

6.5.1.4 On intersubstitutability of trinitarian identity
Finally, the intersubstitutability of identicals fails – another positive result in the current context. In particular, one can think of intersubstitutability in the following form, where P is again any predicate (more importantly, any open

---

[17] By demanding more than just that the pair of claims be either true together or false together, one can get stronger biconditionals than logic's biconditional; however, the idea under discussion is that the power of the trinity rests on the weakness of the logical biconditional that defines trinitarian identity in the usual way.

sentence), a and b any names, and, as above, $\vdash_\Theta$ is the target theological consequence relation:[18]

$$a \simeq b, Pa \nvdash_\Theta Pb$$

That this fails is nicely accounted for by the corresponding failure of detachment for the FDE biconditional (where $\vdash$ is logical consequence):

$$Pa, Pa \leftrightarrow Pb \nvdash Pb$$

A counterexample is a logical possibility in which Pa is a glut and Pb just-false (or Pb is gappy). Such counterexamples can be ruled out as theoretical possibilities, but not in the true theology if, as I've argued, the true theology is contradictory (i.e., glutty). In turn, the invalidity of the corresponding inter-substitutability of trinitarian identicals is likewise refuted by the theological possibility of Christ's contradictory being.

6.5.2 Counting by trinitarian identity

As above, the natural FDE-driven account of trinitarian identity has suffi-cient weakness so as to accommodate at least some of the core trinitarian-identity behavior in a natural and independently motivated way. But what about the *counting* task? What are the proposed 'ways of counting' with respect to trinitarian identity, so understood?

Here, the answer takes a familiar form, although, being in a weaker logical setting, the forms exhibit different behavior from stronger-logical accounts. In particular, letting '$\mathfrak{g}$', '$\mathfrak{f}$', '$\mathfrak{s}$' and '$\mathfrak{h}$' abbreviate (or otherwise stand in for) 'God', 'Father', 'Son' and 'Holy Spirit', respectively, the counting convention may be given as follows, where $\wedge$ is logical conjunction:

- Identity of the *One* god (viz., God): $\mathfrak{g} \simeq \mathfrak{f} \wedge \mathfrak{g} \simeq \mathfrak{s} \wedge \mathfrak{g} \simeq \mathfrak{h}$.[19]
- Non-identity of the *Three* who are God: $\mathfrak{f} \not\simeq \mathfrak{s} \wedge \mathfrak{s} \not\simeq \mathfrak{h} \wedge \mathfrak{h} \not\simeq \mathfrak{f}$.

[18] There are slightly more involved statements of the property but the following suffices for present purposes.

[19] 'There is one god (viz., God)' uses logical quantifiers explicitly, namely, the existential quantifier (i.e., 'there exists an x such that ...'): $\exists x(x \simeq \mathfrak{g} \wedge x \simeq \mathfrak{f} \wedge x \simeq \mathfrak{s} \wedge x \simeq \mathfrak{h})$, though the trinitarian-identity relation itself is defined, per §6.5, via second-order quantification over the target set of properties. In FDE the existential and universal quantifiers are defined standardly (but, of course, do not rule out gluts or gaps). In effect, the existential quantifier behaves like logical disjunction while the universal quantifier behaves like logical conjunction – *like* but not exactly like (but like enough for present purposes). For details see Beall and Logan 2017.

These are the core claims stamped in the Chalcedon-constrained theological tradition; they are the core claims marking the striking fact reflected in the extraordinary trinity: namely, the genuine identity of subjects who are genuinely different – genuine identity despite genuine differences, genuine difference despite genuine identity. The pressing question is how to explain the truth of such core claims on the current contradictory (i.e., glut-theoretic) proposal.

6.5.3   Explanation: gluts from difference

The foregoing approach to trinitarian identity is the obvious first-step account: just invoke the standard story of predicates being true (false) of pairs of objects, and underwrite the claim with the material conditional from logic. In the current context, this account immediately achieves the desideratum of non-transitivity (and, for that matter, also failure of intersubstitutability). But do the key trinitarian-identity claims come out true on this account?

Here, details matter. And the details that matter are exactly the ones that demand a much longer (and deeper) discussion than this chapter (or book) can afford. One of the most pressing issues is how to think of God's properties vis-à-vis the properties of the Father, the Son, and the Spirit, each of whom is (the one and only) God.[20] To avoid complications, and simply to illustrate some of the key issues involved in a glut-theoretic account of trinitarian identity, I pursue a very flat-footed account here: namely, that the properties of God are the pool of properties of the divine persons (viz., Father, Son, Spirit). This immediately raises issues: *But that would mean that God has all the properties of the Father, and the properties of the Son, and all the properties of the Spirit?!* Yes. But as far as I can tell, any explicit account of God's properties vis-à-vis pool of properties of divine persons immediately raises such issues. The issues are important; they are serious; they are difficult. But some such account should be given if one is to give a full account of the trinity, or even of just the relation of trinitarian identity. For present purposes – namely, to just give a sense of some of the issues involved in a glut-theoretic account of the trinity – I select the given flat-footed account and base the discussion on it. Future work must do more.

---

[20] Of course, there's an additional issue that requires treatment in the same project: namely, the simplicity of God in the sense of divine simplicity. For present purposes, I set this aside, using, as throughout the book, 'properties' in the least substantive fashion: they are (at least) whatever is attributed to an entity by a predicate that's true of the given entity.

** *Parenthetical remark.* There are a few other obvious options for answering the question about God's properties vis-à-vis the pool of properties of divine persons. One option is to say that God has none of those properties. In addition to committing heresy-by-omission (e.g., at least if 'person' or 'divine' are properties that must, on pain of heresy-by-omission, be properties of God in the true theology), this no-properties approach puts an immediate stop to the standard first-step approach towards trinitarian identity (since the given biconditionals will one and all be either gappy or just-false, since the divine persons have properties). Another option is to follow a sort of 'dominant' principle, whereby God has those but only those properties that are dominant (so to speak) among the persons – that is, whichever properties are exemplified by at least two of the three divine persons. This option has promise but, at least on the first-step approach towards trinitarian identity at issue, doesn't substantially differ from the flat-footed approach that I adopt for purposes of the current discussion. Variations on these two options are worthy of exploration too. (And this is all in the context of just the first-step approach towards trinitarian identity. There are many different approaches, closely related or otherwise, that must be explored – including but in no way limited to relying on different conditionals in the definition of the identity relation.) *End remark.* **

6.5.3.1 Charting properties

The evaluation (and explanation) of the truth or falsity of the key trinitarian-identity claims turns on the evaluation (and explanation) of the truth or falsity of the target biconditionals. Ignoring the possibility of predicates that are gappy with respect to God (the Father, the Son, the Spirit), I focus on a few predicates that are exemplified by all divine persons (e.g., 'person', 'sinless', 'divine'), some predicates that reflect difference among divine persons (e.g., 'begotten', 'proceeding via Son'), and some that, on Contradictory Christology, are threaded tightly around Christ in a way that reflects his contradictory 2-natured being (e.g., 'human', 'peccable'). I present these in simple charts, each reflecting elements of the unique identical-and-different feature of the trinity.

For convenience, I use 't' and 'f' to indicate that a predicate is just-true and, respectively, just-false of the given subject, and I use 'b' to indicate that the predicate is true and false (i.e., glutty) with respect to the given subject, where subjects (viz., God, Father, Son, Spirit) are listed vertically in the leftmost column, the target predicates horizontally in the top row, and the status of the predicate with respect to the given subject is listed under the predicate in the subject's given row. Example:

	Person	Sinless	Divine
f̵	t	t	t
ȣ̵	t	t	t
ħ	t	t	t
ɡ	t	t	t

Note that without any marked difference in properties, the flat-footed account of God's properties vis-à-vis the properties of divine persons is straightforward, as are the corresponding biconditionals:

- Person($ɡ$) ↔ Person($f̵$)　:　just true.
- Sinless($ɡ$) ↔ Sinless($f̵$)　:　just true.
- Divine($ɡ$) ↔ Divine($f̵$)　:　just true.

And exactly the same, mutatis mutandis, for the Son and Spirit (replacing 'f̵' above with 'ȣ̵' and 'ħ', respectively). Hence, on this restricted picture, there's no hint of God's being glutty (or Christ's being glutty). Restricting just to the given three properties, the important identity claim is entailed:

$$\text{ɡ} \simeq \text{f̵}$$

And the same, in this case, holds for the Son and the Spirit. But, of course, if these were the only properties relevant to the key trinitarian-identity claims then the account commits an unacceptable heresy of omission:[21] the key *difference* among divine persons is *just-false*, that is, the key non-identity claim among persons, namely,

$$\text{f̵} \not\simeq \text{ȣ̵} \wedge \text{ȣ̵} \not\simeq \text{ħ} \wedge \text{ħ} \not\simeq \text{f̵}$$

cannot be in the theory on pain of something just-false being in the theory.

Of course, there is no suggestion that 'person', 'sinless' and 'divine' are the only relevant predicates of divine persons that the true and full theory of the trinity must accommodate; the chart above is used only to illustrate some of the issues on the table. The real hint of trinitarian contradiction arises

---

[21] I should note that, per §4, I truly believe that the substance and sincere aim of genuine heresy is that of omission rather than the appearance of commission – more on which below.

from *differences* among the divine persons, all of whom are *identical* to God. One way of illustrating this is to focus on Christ's contradictory being, and the properties that entail the contradiction, but the real hint of trinitarian contradiction arises from any difference in properties – differences independent from Christ's specific contradictory properties. Consider, in particular, the predicates 'begotten' and 'proceeding via Son', the former true of Christ (indeed, just-true) and no other divine person, the latter true of the Spirit (indeed, just-true) and no other divine person:[22]

	Person	Sinless	Divine	Begotten	Pro-via-$\mathfrak{s}$
$\mathfrak{f}$	t	t	t	f	f
$\mathfrak{s}$	t	t	t	t	f
$\mathfrak{h}$	t	t	t	f	t
$\mathfrak{g}$	t	t	t	?	?

The core of trinitarian contradictions, on the running account, resides in the *differences* among the divine persons *each of whom is identical to the one and only God.* This is the central idea.

The issue of key trinitarian *identities* is now pressing – not surprisingly, given that charted differences above are genuine differences among subjects all of whom are identical to God. The issue is illustrated via the chart's question marks. On this issue, consider the two salient options for question marks:

- Fill in the question marks with either t or f and the required biconditionals fail to deliver the key trinitarian-identity claim:

$$\mathfrak{g} \simeq \mathfrak{f} \wedge \mathfrak{g} \simeq \mathfrak{s} \wedge \mathfrak{g} \simeq \mathfrak{h}$$

  This key truth of the trinity – key trinitarian-identity truth – is *just-false* if 'begotten' is either just-true or just-false of God. (Likewise, mutatis mutandis, for 'proceeds-via-Son'.)

- Fill in the question marks with b.

The latter option is the flat-footed option that I am pursuing: the triune God is contradictory in virtue of exemplifying the pool of properties – including the (so to speak) difference makers – exemplified by all divine persons:

---

[22] Again, if 'proceeding via Son' is not a sufficiently clear case, use any other predicate distinctive of the Spirit. (Again, predicates drawn, e.g., from John 16:7 might do.)

	Person	Sinless	Divine	Begotten	Pro-via-ꝸ
f̄	t	t	t	f	f
ꝸ	t	t	t	t	f
ħ	t	t	t	f	t
g	t	t	t	b	b

This flat-footed account of God's properties affords consistency (i.e., a non-contradictory account) for the Father and the Spirit, and accommodates the independently contradictory case of Christ. And adding Christ's peculiar properties doesn't affect the trinitarian-driven contradictions true of God; they just add to the fuller picture:

	Person	Sinless	Divine	Begotten	Pro-via-ꝸ	Human	Peccable
f̄	t	t	t	f	f	f	f
ꝸ	t	t	t	t	f	t	b
ħ	t	t	t	f	t	f	f
g	t	t	t	b	b	b	b

So goes the flat-footed approach to God's properties. The question is how the approach does with respect to the principal aim: namely, the key trinitarian claims.

6.5.3.2 Key trinitarian identities and non-identities

With God's trinitarian-driven contradictions, as understood above, the key trinitarian identities, which underwrite the *One God*, are all at least true:

- Identity of the *One*: $g \simeq f̄ \wedge g \simeq ꝸ \wedge g \simeq ħ$.

This is true because, for each of the given predicates, there's no pair of the given subjects such that the predicate is neither (at least) true of both nor (at least) false of both, and hence the defining biconditionals are thereby at least true. Moreover, and equally pressing, the corresponding trinitarian non-identities, which underwrite the *Three Persons*,

- Difference of the *Three*: $f̄ \not\simeq ꝸ \wedge ꝸ \not\simeq ħ \wedge ħ \not\simeq f̄$.

This is also true – indeed, just-true – because there are some predicates (e.g., 'begotten', 'proceeds via Son'), illustrated above, that are just-true (just-false) of exactly one of the given subjects (viz., the divine persons).

This much, I believe, is a very promising result from the simple twofold starting point, namely,

- the flat-footed approach to the properties of the one and only (triune) god (viz., God) vis-à-vis the difference-making properties of the Father, Son and Spirit, each of whom is identical to God (the one and only god);
- the first-step approach to the trinitarian-identity relation itself, namely, taking identity claims to be (universally quantified) claims about a set of properties: namely, that the given set of predicates in question are all either at least true of both objects or at least false of both objects in question.

By my lights, this is a very natural and remarkably simple account of trinitarian identity that sits very well with the contradictory truth of Christ.

6.6 The big picture

While the foregoing account naturally and simply delivers the key identity claims and equally key non-identity claims, and does so in a principled fashion, the cost of precision is that all consequences may be seen, even ones that appear to be initially awkward or worse. One key example of this is that in addition to the central claim of God's being the one and only God (i.e., identical with any divine being), namely,

$$g \simeq f \wedge g \simeq \mathsf{s} \wedge g \simeq \mathfrak{h}$$

the difference-making properties (i.e., differences in 't's and 'f's, so to speak) are also properties of God, and so the theory also contains the negation of the given claim, namely,

$$\neg(g \simeq f \wedge g \simeq \mathsf{s} \wedge g \simeq \mathfrak{h})$$

which, by logic, is equivalent to the following disjunction

$$g \not\simeq f \vee g \not\simeq \mathsf{s} \vee g \not\simeq \mathfrak{h}$$

which, in English, amounts to the following claim:

- Either it's false that God is identical to the Father, or it's false that God is identical to the Son, or it's false that God is identical to the Spirit.

Indeed, as a bit of reflection shows, because God is a contradictory being, each such disjunct itself is true (but, notably, each is also false). And this, one might respond, looks like we've clearly crashed an otherwise promising approach. But this response is too quick.[23]

In some (many?) ways, reflection on the trinity should've long ago primed an otherwise unexpected expectation: we should *expect* to have the truth of trinitarian identities only by way of their falsity. After all, the apparent contradiction of the trinity arises exactly from the *identity* of the one and only God despite – or, more accurately, in virtue of – clear and present *differences* in the Three and only three persons each of whom *is identical to* the one and only God. Why should you expect there to be such a reality except in virtue of contradiction?

Accounts of the trinity face the challenge of precisely defining the trinitarian identity relation while – and here is the rub – accommodating the genuine differences among anyone who is identical to the one and only God. If the account of trinitarian identity is sufficiently precise, it's difficult to see how the key truths of the trinity avoid contradictory truths of God. Of course, if the would-be relation of trinitarian identity is simply metaphorical or analogical or anything less than the literal truth of God – one of two truths that distinguish the christian account of God from traditional monotheistic cousins – then contradiction can as easily be avoided as it can be easily disguised or easily equivocated away. My view is that the trinity, and the relation that underwrites it, are not metaphors or analogies; they are essential elements of the truth (the literal truth) of God – contradictory as the truth may be.

On the current proposal, the remarkable trinity of *identical but distinct* subjects – namely, each identical to God and each distinct from the other – is achieved, as with the extraordinary incarnation, via contradiction. The falsity of some key identity claims in no way takes away their truth – an important point that cannot be overemphasized. In particular, it is true –

---

[23] I am, quite sincerely, reminded of a scene in an American pop film that long ago enjoyed mainstream popularity, namely, *Back to the Future*, where, in response to Marty McFly's despondent expression of apparent failure, the scientist Doc Brown replied with the critical and true observation, 'You are not thinking 4-dimensionally.' The current theological issue has nothing to do with thinking 4-dimensionally; however, it may require thinking beyond the standard box.

true, true, true – that the Father is God, the Son (viz., Jesus) is God, and the Holy Spirit is God; the fact that each such claim is also false does not in any way whatsoever undermine its truth; the falsity of the claim simply records more of the extraordinarily rich and unique reality of the trinity.

I am far from convinced that we should reject the given account, wherein the truth of the unique trinity intimately involves falsity, with the given falsity emerging exactly where one would expect – differences among beings each of whom is identical to the one and only God. As above, in many ways this is what we should've expected all along: different entities all of whom are identical to a unique being (viz., God) is fully achieved only via contradiction, and anything less than contradiction yields less than full identity and difference – an identity without a difference, so to speak, or a difference without identity.

Obviously, there is so much more to say, but the more is for future work.

Bibliography

Adams, Marilyn McCord (2006). *Christ and Horrors: The Coherence of Christology*. Cambridge University Press.

Anatolios, Khaled (2011). *Retrieving Nicaea: The Development and Meaning of Trinitarian Doctrine*. Baker Academic, Grand Rapids, MI.

Anderson, Alan Ross and Belnap, Nuel D. (1975). *Entailment: The Logic of Relevance and Necessity*, Volume 1. Princeton University Press, Princeton.

Anderson, Alan Ross, Belnap, Nuel D., and Dunn, J. Michael (1992). *Entailment: The Logic of Relevance and Necessity*, Volume 2. Princeton University Press, Princeton.

Anderson, James (2007). *Paradoxes in Christian Theology*. Paternoster, Waynesboro, GA.

Asenjo, F. G. (1966). A calculus of antinomies. *Notre Dame Journal of Formal Logic*, **7**(1), 103–105.

Asenjo, F. G. and Tamburino, J. (1975). Logic of antinomies. *Notre Dame Journal of Formal Logic*, **16**(1), 17–44.

Ayres, Lewis (2004). *Nicaea and Its Legacy: An Approach to Fourth-Century Trinitarian Theology*. Oxford University Press, New York.

Baber, H. E. (2015). The trinity: Relative identity a redux. *Faith and Philosophy*, **32**(2), 161–171.

Barnes, Michel René (1998). The fourth century as trinitarian canon. In *Christian Origins: Theology, Rhetoric, and Community* (ed. L. Ayres and G. Jones), pp. 47–67. Routledge, London.

Beall, Jc (2000). On truthmakers for negative truths. *Australasian Journal of Philosophy*, **78**(2), 264–268.

Beall, Jc (2004). True and false—as if. In *The Law of Non-Contradiction* (ed. G. Priest, J. Beall, and B. Armour-Garb), pp. 197–216. Oxford University Press, Oxford.

Beall, Jc (2009). *Spandrels of Truth*. Oxford University Press, Oxford.

Beall, Jc (2013a). LP$^+$, K3$^+$, FDE$^+$ and their classical collapse. *Review of Symbolic Logic*, **6**(4), 742–754.

Beall, Jc (2013b). Shrieking against gluts: the solution to the 'just true' problem. *Analysis*, **73**(3), 438–445.

Beall, Jc (2013c). A simple approach towards recapturing consistent theories in paraconsistent settings. *Review of Symbolic Logic*, **6**(4), 755–764.

Beall, Jc (2015). Free of detachment: Logic, rationality, and gluts. *Noûs*, **49**(2), 410–423.

Beall, Jc (2017). There is no logical negation: true, false, both and neither. In *Non-classicality: Logic, Philosophy, and Mathematics* (ed. P. Girarad and Z. Weber). Australasian Journal of Logic, Wellington.

Beall, Jc (2018). The simple argument for subclassical logic. *Philosophical Issues*, **28**(1), 30–54.

Beall, Jc (2019*a*). Christ – a contradiction. *Journal of Analytic Theology*, 7, 400–433.

Beall, Jc (2019*b*). Transparent truth as a logical property. In *The Nature of Truth: Classical and Contemporary Perspectives* (ed. M. P. Lynch, J. Wyatt, J. Kim, and N. Kellen). MIT Press.

Beall, Jc and Burgess, John P. (2017). Logic. In *Oxford Bibliographies* (ed. D. Pritchard). Oxford University Press, Oxford. Online at: https://tinyurl.com/y6zkycgo.

Beall, Jc and Cotnoir, A. J. (2017). God of the gaps: A neglected reply to God's stone problem. *Analysis*, **77**(4), 681–689.

Beall, Jc and Henderson, Jared (2019). A neglected qua solution to the fundamental problem of christology. *Faith and Philosophy*, **36**(2), 157–172.

Beall, Jc and Logan, Shay (2017). *Logic: The Basics* (2nd edn). Routledge, Oxford. First published in 2010.

Beall, J. and Ripley, D. (2004). Analetheism and dialetheism. *Analysis*, **64**(1), 30–35.

Beall, Jc, Pawl, Timothy, McCall, Thomas, Cotnoir, A. J., and Uckelman, Sara L. (2019). Complete symposium on Beall 2019*a*. *Journal of Analytic Theology*, **7**(1), 400–577.

Belnap, N. D. (1977). A useful four-valued logic. In *Modern Uses of Multiple-Valued Logic* (ed. J. M. Dunn and G. Epstein). D. Reidel.

Brower, Jeffrey E. and Rea, Michael C. (2005). Material constitution and the Trinity. *Faith and Philosophy*, **22**(1), 57–76.

Charry, Ellen T. (1997). *By the Renewing of Your Minds: The Pastoral Function of Christian Doctrine*. Oxford University Press, Oxford.

Coakley, Sarah (1999). 'Persons' and the 'social' doctrine of the Trinity: A critique of current analytic discussion. In *The Trinity* (ed. S. T. Davis, D. Kendall, and G. O'Collins), pp. 123–144. Oxford University Press, New York.

Coakley, Sarah (2002). What Chalcedon solved and didn't solve. In *The Incarnation* (ed. S. T. Davis, S. Daniel Kendall, and S. Gerald O'Collins), pp. 143–163. Oxford University Press, Oxford.

Coakley, Sarah (ed.) (2004). *Re-Thinking Gregory of Nyssa*. Blackwell, Oxford.

Coakley, Sarah (2013). *Sexuality and the Self: An Essay 'On the Trinity'*. Cambridge University Press, Cambridge.

Cotnoir, A. J. (2018*a*). Logical nihilism. In *Pluralisms in Truth and Logic* (ed. N. Kellen, N. Pedersen, and J. Wyatt), pp. 301–329. Palgrave Macmillan.

Cotnoir, A. J. (2018*b*). Theism and dialetheism. *Australasian Journal of Philosophy*, **96**(3), 592–609.

Cotnoir, A. J. (2019). On the role of logic in analytic theology: Exploring the wider context of Beall's philosophy of logic. *Journal of Analytic Theology*, **7**(1), 508–528.

Crisp, Oliver D. (2007). *Divinity and Humanity: The Incarnation Reconsidered*. Cambridge University Press, Cambridge, UK.

Crisp, Oliver D. (2009). *God Incarnate: Explorations in Christology*. T & T Clark, New York.

Crisp, Oliver D. and Rea, Michael C. (ed.) (2009). *Analytic Theology: New Essays in the Philosophy of Theology*. Oxford University Press.

Crisp, Oliver D. and Sanders, Fred (ed.) (2014). *Advancing the Trinity: Explorations in Constructive Dogmatics*. Los Angeles Theology Conference Series. Zondervan Academic, Grand Rapids.

Cross, Richard (2002a). *The Metaphysics of the Incarnation: Thomas Aquinas to Duns Scotus*. Oxford University Press UK.

Cross, Richard (2002b). Two models of the Trinity? *Heythrop Journal*, 43(3), 275–294.

Cross, Richard (2011). The incarnation. In *Oxford Handbook of Philosophical Theology* (ed. T. P. Flint and M. Rea). Oxford University Press, Oxford.

Cross, Richard (2019). *Communicatio Idiomatum: Reformation Christological Debates*. Oxford University Press, Oxford.

Dahms, John V. (1978). How reliable is logic? *Journal of the Evangelical Theological Society*, 21(4), 369–380.

Daley, Brian E. (2018). *God Visible: Patristic Christology Reconsidered*. Oxford University Press, Oxford.

Dunn, Geoffrey D. (2001). Divine impassibility and christology in the christmas homilies of Leo the Great. *Theological Studies*, 62(1), 71–85.

Dunn, J. Michael (1966). *The Algebra of Intensional Logics*. Ph.D. thesis, University of Pittsburgh.

Dunn, J. Michael (1976). Intuitive semantics for first-degree entailments and 'coupled trees'. *Philosophical Studies*, 29, 149–168.

Eschenauer Chow, Dawn (2018). The possibility of God. *Faith and Philosophy*, 35(4), 389–407.

Evans, C. S. (1989). Is Kierkegaard an irrationalist? reason, paradox, and faith. *Religious Studies*, 25(3), 347–362.

Ficara, Elena (2009). Der ontologische gottesbeweis bei Hegel und in der analytischen philosophie. In *Gott in der klassischen deutschen Philosophie und im Denken der Gegenwart* (ed. C. Asmuth and K. Drilo), pp. 171–180. Mohr Siebreck, Tübingen.

Field, Hartry (2008). *Saving Truth from Paradox*. Oxford University Press, Oxford.

Fine, Kit (1975). Vagueness, truth and logic. *Synthese*, 30, 265–300.

Flanagan, Owen J. (1991). Consciousness. In *The Science of the Mind* (ed. O. J. Flanagan). MIT Press.

Flanagan, Owen J. (1992). *Consciousness Reconsidered*. MIT Press.

French, Rohan (2016). Structural reflexivity and the paradoxes of self-reference. *Ergo: An Open Access Journal of Philosophy*, 3.

Geach, Peter (1980). *Reference and Generality* (3rd edn). Cornell University Press, Ithaca NY. First edition published 1962.

Gorman, Michael (2016). Classical theism, classical anthropology, and the christological coherence problem. *Faith and Philosophy*, 33(3), 278–292.

Gupta, Anil and Belnap, Nuel (1993). *The Revision Theory of Truth*. MIT Press.

Harman, Gilbert (1986). *Change in View: Principles of Reasoning*. MIT Press, Cambridge, MA.

Harman, Gilbert (1999). Rationality. In *Reasoning, meaning, and mind*, pp. 9–45. Oxford University Press, Oxford.

Hart, Trevor (1995). Sinlessness and moral responsibility: a problem in christology. *Scottish Journal of Theology*, 38, 37–54.

Holmes, Stephen R. (2012). *The Quest for the Trinity: The Doctrine of God in Scripture, History and Modernity*. IVP Academic, Downers Grove, IL.

Jedwab, Joseph (2015). Against the Geachian theory of the Trinity and incarnation. *Faith and Philosophy*, **32**(2), 125–145.

Leftow, Brian (2002). A timeless god incarnate. In *The Incarnation* (ed. S. T. Davis, D. Kendall, and G. O'Collins), pp. 273–99. Oxford University Press, Oxford.

Lehmann, Helmut T. (ed.) (1971). *Luther's Works: Word and Sacrament*, Volume 4. Fortress Press, Minneapolis, MN.

Lewis, David K. (1975). Languages and language. In *Minnesota Studies in the Philosophy of Science* (ed. K. Gunderson), pp. 3–35. University of Minnesota Press. Reprinted in (Lewis, 1983).

Lewis, David K. (1983). *Philosophical Papers*, Volume I. Oxford University Press, Oxford.

Lewis, David K. (1986). *On the Plurality of Worlds*. Wiley-Blackwell.

Martinich, A. P. (1978). Identity and Trinity. *Journal of Religion*, **58**(2), 169–181.

Martinich, A. P. (1979). God, emperor, and relative identity. *Franciscan Studies*, **39**, 180–191.

Maudlin, Tim (2004). *Truth and Paradox: Solving the Riddles*. Oxford University Press.

McCall, Thomas H. (2010). *Which Trinity? Whose Monotheism?: Philosophical and Systematic Theologians on the Metaphysics of Trinitarian Theology*. W.B. Eerdmans Pub. Co.

McCall, Thomas H. (2015). *An Invitation to Analytic Christian Theology*. InterVarsity Academic Press.

McCall, Thomas H. (2019). Doctrinal orthodoxy and philosophical heresy: A theologian's reflections on Beall's proposal. *Journal of Analytic Theology*, **7**, 473–487.

McCall, Thomas H. and Rea, Michael C. (ed.) (2009). *Philosophical and Theological Essays on the Trinity*. Oxford University Press, Oxford.

McGinn, Colin (1991). *The Problem of Consciousness: Essays Toward a Resolution*. Blackwell.

Meyer, Robert K. (1971). Entailment. *Journal of Philosophy*, **68**(21), 808–818.

Morris, Thomas V. (1986). *The Logic of God Incarnate*. Ithaca: Cornell University Press.

Nagasawa, Yujin (2008). A new defence of Anselmian theism. *Philosophical Quarterly*, **58**(233), 577–596.

Nagasawa, Yujin (2017). *Maximal God: A New Defence of Perfect Being Theism*. Oxford University Press.

Pawl, Timothy (2014). A solution to the fundamental philosophical problem of christology. *Journal of Analytic Theology*, **2**, 61–85.

Pawl, Timothy (2016). *In Defense of Conciliar Christology: A Philosophical Essay*. Oxford University Press, Oxford.

Pawl, Timothy (2019a). Explosive theology. *Journal of Analytic Theology*, **7**(1), 440–451.

Pawl, Timothy (2019b). *In Defense of Extended Conciliar Christology: A Philosophical Essay*. Oxford University Press, Oxford.

Pawl, Timothy (2020). *Incarnation*. Cambridge University Press, Cambridge.

Plantinga, Alvin (1983). Reason and belief in God. In *Faith and Rationality: Reason and Belief in God* (ed. A. Plantinga and N. Wolterstorff), pp. 16–93. University of Notre Dame Press.

Plantinga, Alvin (2000). *Warranted Christian Belief*. Oxford University Press, USA.

Pleitz, Martin (2015). Priest and the holy Trinity. Slides: presented at a Münseter workshop on Graham Priest's metaphysics monograph *One*.

Priest, Graham (1979). The logic of paradox. *Journal of Philosophical Logic*, **8**, 219–241.

Priest, Graham (1998). To be and not to be – that is the answer. on Aristotle on the law of non-contradiction. *Logical Analysis and History of Philosophy*, **1**, 91–130.

Priest, Graham (2000). Motivations for paraconsistency: The slippery slope from classical logic to dialetheism. In *Frontiers of Paraconsistency* (ed. D. Batens, C. Mortensen, G. Priest, and J.-P. V. Bendegem). Research Studies Press, King's College Publications, Baldock.

Priest, Graham (2006). *In Contradiction* (Second edn). Oxford University Press, Oxford. First printed by Martinus Nijhoff in 1987.

Priest, Graham (2014). *One: Being an Investigation into the Unity of Reality and of its Parts, Including the Singular Object Which Is Nothingness*. Oxford University Press.

Priest, Graham, Beall, Jc, and Armour-Garb, B. (ed.) (2004). *The Law of Non-Contradiction*. Oxford University Press, Oxford.

Quine, W. V. (1969). Epistemology naturalized. In *Ontological Relativity and Other Essays*. New York: Columbia University Press.

Rea, Michael C. (2003). Relative identity and the doctrine of the Trinity. *Philosophia Christi*, **5**(2), 431–445.

Rea, Michael C. (2011). The Trinity. In *Oxford Handbook of Philosophical Theology* (ed. T. P. Flint and M. Rea). Oxford University Press, Oxford.

Rea, Michael C. (2014). *Metaphysics: The Basics*. Routledge.

Rojek, Paweł (2019). Pavel Florensky's theory of religious antinomies. *Logica Universalis*, **13**(4), 515–540.

Routley, Richard (1979). Dialectical logic, semantics and metamathematics. *Erkenntnis*, **14**, 301–331.

Routley, Richard and Meyer, Robert K. (1976). Dialectical logic, classical logic, and the consistency of the world. *Studies in East European Thought*, **16**(1–2), 1–25.

Routley, Richard, Plumwood, Val, Meyer, Robert K., and Brady, Ross T. (ed.) (1982). *Relevant Logics and their Rivals*. Ridgeview.

Russell, Gillian (2018). Logical nihilism: Could there be no logic? *Philosophical Issues*, **28**(1), 308–324.

Senor, Thomas D. (2002). Incarnation, timelessness, and Leibniz's Law problems. In *God and Time: Essays on the Divine Nature* (ed. G. E. Ganssle and D. M. Woodruff). Oxford University Press.

Shapiro, Stewart (1991). *Foundations Without Foundationalism: A Case for Second-Order Logic*. Oxford University Press, Oxford.

Stump, Eleonore (2003). *Aquinas*. Routledge.

Swinburne, Richard (1994). *The Christian God*. Oxford University Press.

Tanner, Norman P. (1990). *Decrees of the Ecumenical Councils (2 volume set)*. Georgetown University Press.

Tarski, Alfred (1956). *Logic, Semantics, Metamathematics: Papers from 1923 to 1938*. Clarendon Press, Oxford. Translated by J. H. Woodger.

Tertullian, I. (1956). *Treatise on the Incarnation*. SPCK, London. Trans. by Ernest Evans.

Torrance, Andrew (2019). The possibility of a scientific approach to analytic theology. *Journal of Analytic Theology*, 7(1), 178–198.

Torrance, Andrew (2020). Kierkegaard's paradoxical theology. *Participatio*, 5, 60–81. Published in the supplemental volume of the Journal: Sören Kierkegaard as a Christian, Incarnational Theologian.

Tuggy, Dale (2009). Paradox in Christian theology: An analysis of its presence, character, and epistemic status. *Faith and Philosophy*, 26(1), 104–108.

Tuggy, Dale (2011). On positive mysterianism. *International Journal for Philosophy of Religion*, 69(3), 205–226.

Tuggy, Dale (2016). Trinity. In *The Stanford Encyclopedia of Philosophy* (Winter 2016 edn) (ed. E. N. Zalta). Metaphysics Research Lab, Stanford University.

Uckelman, Sara L. (2019). Contradictions, impossibility, and triviality: A response to Jc Beall. *Journal of Analytic Theology*, 7(1), 544–559.

van Inwagen, Peter (1988). And Yet They Are Not Three Gods But One God. In *Philosophy and the Christian Faith* (ed. T. V. Morris), Volume 5 of *Notre Dame Studies in the Philosophy of Religion*, pp. 241–278. University of Notre Dame Press.

van Inwagen, Peter (1994). Not by confusion of substance, but by unity of person. In *Reason and the Christian Religion: Essays in Honour of Richard Swinburne* (ed. R. Swinburne and A. G. Padgett). Oxford University Press.

Vohánka, Vlastimil (2013). Why Peter van Inwagen does not help in showing the logical possibility of the Trinity. *Studia Neoaristotelica*, 10(2), 196–214.

Williams, C. J. F. (1968). A programme for christology. *Religious Studies*, 3(2), 513–524.

Wolfson, H. A. (1964). *The Philosophy of the Church Fathers: Faith, Trinity, Incarnation*. Harvard University Press, Cambridge, MA.

Index